MW01233530

FACING AUTISM

FIRST PERSON JOURNEYS OF AUTISM

THE FACING PROJECT PRESS
An imprint of The Facing Project
Muncie, Indiana 47305
facingproject.com

First published in the United States of America by The Facing Project Press, an imprint of The Facing Project and division of The Facing Project Gives Inc., 2022.

First paperback edition March 2022

Cover design by Shantanu Suman

Library of Congress Control Number: 2022933165

ISBN: 978-1-7345581-8-0 (paperback)
ISBN: 978-1-7345581-9-7 (eBook)

Printed in the United States of America

10 9 8 7 6 5 4 3 2 1

CONTENTS

EDITORS' NOTE

In 2013, The Facing Project partnered with multiple organizations to tell the stories of parents, therapists, and children in *Facing Autism in Muncie*. After printing and dispersing 6,000 copies of that book, we have decided to revisit some of those stories, and gather new ones focused on adults with autism.

In the next decade alone, it's estimated that 500,000 teens with autism will age out of school-based services and enter the world as adults. The stories that follow will take you on a journey from adolescence to adulthood, heartbreak to hope, grief to gratitude, and loneliness to love—from learning to drive to determining what college to attend to running a business, these stories are a reminder of the human condition that connects us all.

It's also important to note that The Facing Project collects stories from all walks of life, and we believe that everyone has a story to share. These stories are the storyteller's truth and lived experience, and we acknowledge that every story may not reflect the viewpoints of every reader or that of The Facing Project staff, volunteers, or Board of Directors.

Ultimately, it is our hope that these stories will serve as a resource, offer insights, create conversations, open hearts and minds, and will give you the courage to share your own story and the empathy to listen to others.

Kelsey Timmerman and J.R. Jamison
Co-founders of The Facing Project

1

A WORLD FOR MY KIDS (2021)

BELINDA HUGHES'S STORY AS TOLD TO CHRISTINE RHINE

One day when Gabe was about seven, he was flapping his hands and bouncing on a ball in his room. I told him he could flap his hands but only there, only in his room. I told him, "I'm trying so hard to prepare this world for you. I'm trying so hard."

Today with each clinic we open, each new outreach, I think: *Now I'm preparing this corner of the world for you, and now this corner.* So much has happened since Gabe was little, since he was first diagnosed. Now there's not just a world to prepare for him, there's a world that's making accommodations for him.

It's so rewarding to see the changes and to be a part of that system that is growing, expanding understanding, and teaching so many parents, grandparents, teachers, and friends how to interact and what to expect from a family member with autism. There are ways of responding and ways parents can play with their child, grow closer, really bond.

It was so hard at first. It was hard to find research, to find doctors, experts. I know what it's like to be empty, to be depleted, to be *on* all the time. I've tried to create a community here in Muncie to care for families, parents, grandparents, and to help these children reach for their best lives.

Gabe is twenty-one now. If you'd told me when he was seven what I would go through, where I would be now, I wouldn't have believed you.

"Gabe, do you like being an adult?"

"Yes," Gabe responds, emphatically.

"What's the best thing about being an adult?"

"Man cave."

His man cave is his favorite place. Gabe has his own house now. The man cave is his train room, filled with toy trains and cars. He loves having that freedom. A therapist comes every morning, Monday through Friday, to make sure he showers and makes his breakfast, gets dressed. Then around noon Gabe comes to the clinic I run for children with autism. He does chores which he gets paid for. He loves getting paid! He can use his money to buy more toy cars or something else he wants.

His favorite chore is taking out the trash, which is not what I would have picked for him, but he loves it because he gets to go into every room and talk to everybody. He especially loves it if the bags get heavy and he has to use muscle power to carry them to the dumpster.

The staff, everyone at the clinic, is his family. We have fifty-eight students now and seventy-eight staff. One day when Gabe had experienced some trauma, it took several of them to hold him, to keep him from hurting himself. When he was able to calm down, he started crying. They all started crying, too. As he relaxed, he kept saying, "Thank you, friends, thank you." My heart is happy that he knows he is loved and that he has a whole community around him that loves him, knows him, and is happy to see him.

We have a staff daycare, and the little ones love Gabe. He reads to them. He makes recordings of himself reading Thomas the Train books for them—he reads with a lot of emphasis and drama. The littles love it.

Everyone wants a purpose, to have a life where they have purpose, they contribute, they have joy. That is what I want for my kids. And they're all my kids.

PROUD TO BE A PERSON WITH AUTISM (2021)

MADISON STEVENSON'S STORY AS TOLD TO LIZ BERGREN

I am not through the door yet when I hear, "Good morning, Madison!" from somewhere down the hallway. I smile slightly; glance down at my feet and say, "Good morning."

I rush to catch up with my best friend so we can walk to class together. In a few short weeks, I will be graduating. Of course, I am excited to graduate. I can't wait to go to college. It will be bittersweet, leaving this place. I am comfortable here. It's hard to explain but I have never felt this way about school before. I have always felt out of place. As though I didn't fit. I excelled academically, especially in math, but socially I felt isolated and spent a lot of time alone. The Excel Center is different. It isn't just my school; it feels like home. I can be myself here and not worry about being judged or bullied.

I was four years old when I was diagnosed with autism spectrum disorder. I remember feeling confused and asking my mom a bunch of questions. *Why did I have it? What did it even mean?*

My grandmother told me that she could tell there was something different about me, but I didn't feel different. I felt like me. As I grew older, I started to notice differences between me and other kids. I felt nervous a lot and it was difficult for me to make eye contact or talk to new people. Sometimes, I felt worthless. Like I didn't fit with anyone.

When I was twelve years old, I met two close friends. In school and at camp, we laughed together. I felt the same way around my friends as I did with my mentor, my behavior analyst. I never felt as though I needed to change who I was around them. Over the last six years, our friendships have grown and strengthened. Still, I have days where I feel lonely and uncertain. Sometimes, it is difficult for me to adjust when something doesn't go well or how I planned. In those moments, I know I can turn to my friends and God for understanding.

Close relationships with my family and friends have allowed me to feel valued and understood. My confidence has grown and I no longer feel self-conscious about my disorder or how I choose to cope. Stimming is short for "self-stimulatory behavior." Many people with autism use stimming behaviors to cope when they feel excited or upset. I may rock side to side or rhythmically tap my fingers. Others may pace or rub their hands back and forth. The repetitive movements create a calming sensation. I used to feel as though I needed to hide my stimming. Now, I know that it is just as much a part of me as my smile or my laugh.

In a few weeks, I will graduate high school. A few months after that, I will begin working on a double major in

Nursing and Applied Behavior Analysis at Ball State University, eventually serving in a nursing home or hospital. Some people may see autism spectrum disorder as an obstacle to be overcome. I just see it as part of my story that has many chapters. Chapters like a fun and close relationship with my younger brother. Chapters filled with hopes of having a loving husband and two daughters. I have learned to have confidence in my abilities and to embrace who I am, and I hope to inspire others to do the same.

I am proud to be a person with autism. I consider it a gift that has transformed my life and shaped me into the young woman I am today. If I were given the chance to change anything, I wouldn't. This is who I am.

TACKLE (2013)

CHAD SHELLEY'S STORY AS TOLD TO TOM STEINER

Jackson's heart is unbelievably big. I am most proud that he can see the good in others.

On his first day of kindergarten, a child who wanted Jackson's eyeglasses bullied him. At one point, the child tried to grab them. Jackson held up his hand and said, "No." Eventually the bully did get the glasses and proceeded to break them. But Jackson stood up for himself.

No matter how much we want to be there for Jackson each moment, every day we send him off into a world that we fear is full of bullies and cruel jokes. Often Jackson eases our fears and surprises us with the kindness and love he brings and inspires.

At first there was denial.

Every father thinks his son is going to follow in his own footsteps. My father played college football, I played college football, and now I am going to get to watch my son carry on the tradition. That's what I thought.

I played defensive end. Each play was a solvable problem: the other team was trying to advance the ball; I was the solution. Tackle them. I think a lot of guys are like this. As soon as we're told there's a problem, we want to fix it immediately. When there were concerns that Jackson had developmental delays, my way of facing the problem was thinking, "It's not true; he's just fine. He looks like a typical kid. He's fine."

Every time Allison, my wife, would bring up something about Jackson's early childhood development, I would not want to talk about it. In hindsight, I was not very helpful. At two-years, Jackson was a little more delayed for his age group. He didn't have a large vocabulary, but how large should it be at that age? As the eternal optimist, I just kept thinking: *Everything is fine, there is nothing wrong with Jackson; he'll catch up.*

I was just looking for what I wanted to see. I was comforted by Jackson's smiles when he would run to me, and I would throw him into the air. And I ignored the fact that once I put his feet back on the ground, he rarely made eye contact with anyone.

By the age of three he started to spin around in circles. It was impressive. I took the guy approach once again and would joke around saying Jackson is going to be the toughest ballerina in the world because that kid could pirouette like none other.

When Jackson and I went to the park, I would see other kids his age running around and playing. Jackson would only want to swing and not just for a few moments, we're talking about an hour, two hours straight. I could see the difference in how they played and how he played. I could feel the difference.

Soon he was diagnosed with Pervasive Development Disorder, which is to say, he displays some of the symptoms on the autism spectrum but not all of them. Later that year at Riley Hospital in Indianapolis, the diagnosis would be that Jackson, my future pirouetting football player, was autistic.

I did not want to label him as being autistic. I didn't want to believe it because once I allowed it in my mind, I knew it would become true in my heart. From now on, this is what we were facing and I wanted nothing to do with that. This wasn't a problem you could just tackle.

I did not want to believe my son was on the Autism Spectrum. However, once I admitted it, I could only think about what kind of a life he was going to have now.

I would hold him and rock him to sleep, or I would lay with him in his bed and smell his hair and pray that he would be able to enjoy life and be happy. There were moments where I was disappointed and discouraged, but it was always for him. Not that I wanted him to be an all-star football player, but I just wanted him to have a good life.

Initially my wife and I were on two different islands. Allison was the advocate reading and educating herself. I would come home and the last thing I wanted to do was think about things, about autism. I just wanted to unplug and be at home and enjoy my family.

When I look back now, boy, I was a jerk.

Allison wanted to help our son, and I'm telling her everything is going to be fine. She was fighting for our son; I was standing on the sidelines. I should have been right there with her, as her defensive end.

When I finally got on board and started walking side-by-side with her, it was more about how did Jackson's day go. Was it a huge step back or a great step forward?

Then the biggest stress that autism brought to our family was how to get Jackson what he needed. Early intervention is so important. There's a window until the age of seven where we had to get him everything he needed: therapy, speech therapy, and social groups, whatever it might be. You have to get them involved in everything even though they may fight it.

We understood the battle and the emotional and financial costs; we sacrificed and gave until we hurt.

Parker, our second son, is four. He calls Jackson, Bubba, and thinks he is made out of the moon and the stars. They are best buddies. We could not be happier. Parker has been fantastic; Jackson has looked out for him like a big brother would. Allison and I try to stay very cognizant on giving them equal amount of attention. There are times when it is one sided, but that is unfortunately unavoidable. We try to keep it equal and hold them to the same standards. I think this has helped Jackson become the person he is becoming. He has more challenges than Parker, but we still expect him to do well. As long as he's giving his best, which is what is truly important to us.

Eventually, we figured out that all we could control was how it was going to affect us today. This made life more bearable. I have a partner in Allison who has borne a tremendous amount of that weight and responsibility. I try to be the moral support. She was and still is an incredible voice for Jackson. She is behind the scenes making it all happen, working with him at home.

If I could rewind the clock, it would be that I jumped in

with two feet. Allison did, and she needed someone to jump in with her.

The Real Hero of the Story

Remember that kindergarten bully? Well, a few months after he had bullied Jackson, an older boy was bullying the bully. Jackson got in between the older boy and his class-mate and said, "Quit bullying my friend. That's not nice. Go pick on someone your own size." The older kid turned and walked away.

I wish I had known earlier how much of a fighter Jackson was. He does not know any differently. To him, he just knows, "I have to work my tail off." He has done so well with everything that has been laid out in front of him.

As parents our job is to lead our children, but some-times our children lead us.

I never thought about things this way until the company I work for sent me through the Lead ECI Leadership Training program. During one of the sessions, they asked me to think about the one person who has really impacted my life. I thought of Jackson and the struggles he faces every day. Yet he gets up in the morning with the same amount of enthusiasm to take that day on as he did the day before and the day before that.

I told the group that my son has taught me to never give up. Don't ever think of throwing in that towel.

While telling everyone, I wept. The tears weren't of grief or mourning. They existed at a moment, when this grown man, a former college football player, realized that his young son was his hero.

4

THRIVING IN THE UNKNOWN (2013)

ALLISON SHELLEY'S STORY AS TOLD TO SUZANNE CLEM

I t rocks your world. It really does.

Having a medical background, knowing the milestones a child should be hitting, I knew at one year that things didn't seem quite right. By eighteen months, being around people outside of our home practically paralyzed him. By age two, it wasn't much better. We didn't have a diagnosis, but for me it was already real. I was already grieving the reality that he wasn't going to be the child my husband and I thought he'd be, and I felt like we were wasting valuable time without a diagnosis that could tell us for sure what we were facing.

We finally found ourselves in an appointment at Riley Hospital, and within an hour the doctor put a stop to the frustration of waiting. "Absolutely," he said. "He has autism." When he said it out loud, it was crushing.

All these thoughts go through your head. *He may never speak. He may never be potty-trained. He may never go to school.*

And while the helpless feeling of not being able to decisively say "this is autism" was put to rest in that doctor's appointment, it was replaced with helpless feelings of watching our son struggle, of having to rely on trial and error in the pursuit of medication that would make a meaningful difference, of not knowing how you're supposed to plan for something that is so unknown.

A turning point came for us when we enrolled Jackson in Muncie's then-new ABA clinic—an applied behavioral analysis clinic. Most moms get to wait until their kids are five or six before they send them off to a full day of kindergarten or first grade, but my baby was still three years old and I was sending him off to strangers for eight hours a day. And they were challenging him. Really challenging him. To the point where sometimes I'd push back. He was almost four, but he was my baby. I'd say, "This is too hard for him." Throw into the mix a financial state that's at its low and a new baby on its way, and you come up with a pretty emotionally exhausted family. It was hard. But for Jackson, it was also working. The methods they were using at the clinic were working, and they continued working.

By age six, he had gone from a little boy who couldn't talk, couldn't make eye contact, and wasn't potty-trained to a student ready to graduate from his ABA program and enter a kindergarten classroom—a mainstream public-school classroom, full of neuro-typical children, without the need of an aide. The feeling of joy that brought made it all worth it.

We cherish the joys, while embracing a life that has become a balancing act of accomplishments and struggles. It's an accomplishment for him to thrive in a classroom with peers who can look out for him and help him through unfamiliar situations, but it's a struggle when he gets confused stares and awkward reactions from classmates who don't understand why he's standing so close or why he won't stop talking about video games. It's an accomplishment that he puts his shoes on by himself or gets ready for dinner by himself, but we might later have to explain why it's important that the left shoe go on the left foot and the right shoe on the right foot, or how exactly to turn the water on, grab the soap, lather it, rinse it off your hands, and turn the water off.

The hardest balancing act comes when I see people watching him and know that they see him as "different."

One of my greatest fears is that people aren't going to recognize him for who he is on the inside, focusing only on his outward behaviors. I really have to work to balance my immediate feelings of hurt with the knowledge that if it doesn't bother him, it shouldn't bother me. And there's something to be grateful for there. When someone makes fun of him, he may not quite get it—and if he does, he probably won't care enough to hold on to it and be bothered by it for days. It's a blessing, and it allows him to continue to grow.

At age eight, Jackson is getting to the point where he realizes his experience is different than his classmates' and that things are harder for him than others—he realizes that the math problems that take him hours might take the kid sitting next to him minutes. That the words other students can spell after a couple tries might take him twenty. That's hard for a mom to watch. How do you explain that to a child who's probably worked harder than any other child in his class to get to where he is? How are we going to explain it when his younger brother begins achieving things that he hasn't yet been able to accomplish and might not be able to? That's where we say, "Jackson, it's not fair. It's really not. But this is the hand we're dealt, and we can do the best we can."

Which is exactly what Jackson is doing. He's exceeded so many expectations that we just keep setting the bar higher.

And now? We celebrate now.

This year is the first year he'll have a birthday party with friends he picked out on his own and invited to come. Back in the "dark days," as we called them, we wondered things like: *Will he ever have friends who care about him? Will he ever have friends that he cares about?* To have friends who genuinely want to be his friend and who genuinely like him for who he is . . . it's awesome.

We celebrate his friendships, we celebrate the high-functioning child he's become, and we celebrate the potential that lies in a future unknown but full of possibility. As long as he's finding his place, that's to be celebrated—no matter what.

5

DRIVEN (2021)

ALLISON SHELLEY'S STORY AS TOLD TO CHRIS BAVENDER

Jackson turned sixteen this past Sunday. It blows my mind. I don't know how we got to sixteen. I don't feel old enough to have a sixteen-year-old.

He is a freshman at Muncie Central High School. I was probably a lot more nervous about him going to high school than he was. He is pretty chill about all things all the time. But I was pretty stressed about it.

We knew he would go to high school, but we didn't know what that would look like. But when we had our IEP (individual education plan) meeting to talk about what diploma he would get (in Indiana there are different ones you can get, and Core 40 is the traditional diploma), we were expecting the academic folks to say they wanted him to get the equivalent of a GED, which meant he'd graduate, but really not look to pursue college. But they recommended him for the Core 40. I said, "Are you sure we are talking about the same kid? Are you in the right file? We are talking about Jackson, right?" They said yes, they didn't see any reason he couldn't do it, and I was like: *Who am I to disagree?* We had the biggest celebration.

For so long we have been pushing for him to do more. In the beginning, the school wanted him in special education classes. It would have been easier, but we have pushed a lot over the years to challenge him to rise to the occasion. When we got to high school, we thought we would get pushback from teachers and administrators, but everyone thought he could do it. I remember my husband and I sitting there saying, "Oh, wow, we don't have to fight!" Probably the best and quickest IEP meeting we have had. Usually, we come in ready to fight and advocate for him, and we did not have to this time. So, this is a big deal for him and for us.

It's pretty amazing to me. It's not like I was going to doubt it, but I wasn't sure we would get to the point where we were all on the same page. I wanted it for him, but was prepared for it not to happen.

He takes all the regular classes like biology, Japanese— all the classes neurotypical kids are taking. Some he is doing well in, and some not so well, but I think he is going to do it. He constantly needs to be told to finish things. He will have papers stuffed in his backpack that are half finished—that is the stuff that drives me crazy. I tell him, "You have to work harder than everyone else," and he is just like, "Eh, I will turn it in."

He is a teacher's dream. He sits in the back of class quietly; he doesn't say a bad thing. He is just an easy-going kid. Sometimes I worry that we should be pushing him more. I do push him probably more than anyone else in his life. But I feel like it's a mom's job anyway.

He has a resources study hall instead of a typical study hall. Meaning there is an actual resource teacher in there helping them with their work. Yes, it is a free period, but the only other kids in there are those that also need a little extra help—an extra period to catch up. And an opportunity for someone else to ask why he has eight half-finished pages in biology instead of his mom yelling at him.

Sometimes I just have to walk away. I will say to him, "You're killing me! Not really, but you are, buddy. Why do all this work and not turn it in?" Stuff that makes me crazy. So, I say, "Mom is going to go for a walk, or a run, then come back and help. I just need a minute."

We use a lot of Post-it Notes. We Post-it his notebooks and his Chromebook, as a visual reminder to talk to so-and-so about such-and-such. And he will be very proud, and bring the Post-it Notes home and have written *yes* or checked it off or crossed it off. He will be very proud he took care of it which is great, and we tell him we are proud of him for doing that, but we also really would like to know what the teacher thought.

I think the biggest challenge for him right now is that he is a sixteen-year-old boy and also a sixteen-year-old boy with autism. It's hard to know if the things he is doing are just because he is a sixteen-year-old boy, or because he is a sixteen-year-old boy with autism. That is the biggest struggle.

He is starting driver's ed and he is going to do in-person training with a teacher. He is probably not going to catch on as fast as others, but he is not the first young man on the spectrum they have trained, and they didn't bat an eye.

He's not in a super rush to drive because he is like, *where am I going to go?* School and back. Maybe stop at the gas station and get a Dr. Pepper because that is his favorite thing. But we feel it is a milestone we really want him to achieve—whether he spends a lot of time driving or not—it's just nice to know he could.

I think there is a little bit of stress now as he gets closer to being an adult—a legal adult who will graduate from high school, and we don't know what post-high school looks like for him. Again, I don't know that it is much different than other parents of sixteen-year-olds. If he wants to go to college, he is going to go local, so we are around.

He will kick around ideas of things he would like to do for a job and sometimes I think: *Oh, that would work, that would be feasible.* But other times I don't—but I don't want to dismiss anything. The nice thing about Muncie Central is the option to go to the Muncie Area Career Center and take classes there. We hope something will spark his interest.

Ultimately, we want him to be happy. We want him to find his niche, and be a productive member of society, which I think is the goal of most parents.

He continues to exceed our expectations in every way and—I am not going to cry—but he has worked, and we have worked very hard for it. I am not sure that anyone really knows how hard it is to try to fit in when you know that you don't.

He is a pretty amazing kid.

AND A BLESSING (2021)

JACKSON SHELLEY'S STORY AS TOLD TO CHRIS BAVENDER

I want people to know that what you have is not important, you are gifted just the way you are.

I would say that not only is autism a curse, but it can be a blessing. A curse that you might forget something, but the blessing is you get to do a lot of things that other people don't do—like being a visual learner or learning to read.

School is pretty good. I like social studies because it's about history and geography. I like Japan. I am taking Japanese. You have to write it very neatly; it is very hard. Some things are harder like math; it's not visual.

I like to read books, just subject vs. author, nonfiction or fiction. Monster books—basically the pictures. I also like to read them, too.

One of my friends is Ollie. Sometimes we like to play outside or with Nerf guns. Ollie is like my person at school if I need to talk. He's a very good kid. My other friend is Lucas. I get to eat lunch with him every other day. He is also on the spectrum, and he is really smart and funny. We like some of the same things, and I know that I can just be myself when I am with him. I like lunch better on the days I sit with him. The other days I sit by myself. Which is okay because I am used to it.

But having a friend is better.

I honestly think I might be a chef or a night guard. I make my own stuff. I do like food and food shows. I also like animal shows. Whatever job I do, I know I will work hard at it and do a good job.

ONE DAY, I'LL FLAP MY ARMS IN FREEDOM, AND NO ONE WILL CARE (2021)

KYLE RENINGER'S STORY AS TOLD TO JASON NEWMAN

I was in my mid-twenties when I hit the wall. Amanda and I had been together for about ten years, married for about three, and we were having a rough time. I was depressed, and tired, and I really didn't like what was going on in my life. And one day, we were listening to an NPR story, and they were interviewing this guy that wrote this book: *The Journal of Best Practices*. It was about a guy who started to see, later in life, that he was on the autism spectrum. And we looked at each other like, *Wait a minute!* That's how I started this journey.

Growing up, I never thought I was different. My parents set very clear expectations of what I was supposed to act like in public, so I knew. I ended up dropping out of college, working at Starbucks for a dozen years. I sold TVs and electronics at Circuit City. I've done a lot of those jobs where I'm very people forward. My dad was always a salesman, so I got really good at mimicking those kinds of personas. But then it became too much, working in sales; I started to see all of these different masks I was wearing. There was *work Kyle*, and I have *home Kyle*, and I have *friend Kyle*, and so I was able to compartmentalize everything. Then I started having all of these major depression and anxiety issues, and I realized: *Hey, you can't keep this up your whole life!* It was too draining to be these different people six days a week.

So, I started this journey. I started by taking these online tests, and I'm scoring ninety-three out of a hundred. I'd give them to Amanda, and she'd get like a thirty. So, we knew there was something there. We started doing more research, and it just sort of aligned, and helped explain a lot of the difficulties I've had throughout my life—interacting with people, and myself. What I liked about the research, and like Facebook groups now, is I get to see how a lot of other people took this journey, and how they're doing it. I met people who had been diagnosed when they were little kids, and some who were in their teens. And I started going back and forth: *Is there a right way of doing this journey?* I'm learning about where other people are on their journey, and I'm integrating those people, and stories, into mine.

That's helped, because when I started this journey, I lost a job because of it. I lost friends, because I wasn't the same jolly Kyle they always knew. So, that was difficult. But it was also really freeing in a lot of ways. Now that I know, I have a lot fewer major depressive or anxiety attacks. I still get them, but not the major ones, and not every day. Now I build in the wind down time I need during the day, or after work. I know how to decompress; a lot of television, games, or screen time. And now, I can be very helpful to the business because I love the delivery time where I can just drive and listen to podcasts and have that alone time that I need.

It's helped because I've started, you know, to kind of help Amanda be more like me, and she's helped me be more like her. Like the other night, we're lying in bed, and I say, "Hey why don't we take our dogs for a walk?" And she's like, "What? That's not our routine," and I was thinking that we needed to get up and be active, and out of our routine. So, we're getting closer because of that. I'm learning to be a better man because I'm learning how my brain works. Like, I'm really good with systems, creating them, playing with them, making them better. So, now, I can find the things that really come easy for me.

A lot of stereotypes of autistic people is that we're loners, and that we want to be alone. And that may be, for some, but I think it's more that social interaction is difficult for us. I see a lot of really lonely people, reaching out to make connections. So, I think, learning this about me later in life, helped me. I already had that connection with Amanda. A lot of people learn when they're kids, and are told they can't, so they don't. I see a lot of us struggling with stimming in public. You know, some things are okay to do. But I look for the day that I can flap my arms in freedom, and no one cares.

All of us autistics are different. I want to learn what I'm like, and learn what you're like so we can express ourselves better. So, I'm here, telling my story. I want to add my vegetables to this stew, and cook yours in too.

HEALING IS BELIEVING (2013)

ANGELA'S STORY AS TOLD TO KELSEY TIMMERMAN

The circus curtains in the boys' room were iridescent. They were beautiful. I wanted to burn them.

The fabric represented such sadness, such a loss, such a complete disaster. I wanted to reclaim the space in a different way. Get rid of all that stuff and start from scratch. I donated them, giving them a chance to be transformed into something happier, to be repurposed.

————

In many ways our story is one of transformation. When I tell it, I usually lose people. Let's just say that I know what the "glaze over" looks like.

Our story is so much bigger than vaccinations, but that's where it began six years ago.

At eight months, our son Peter was smiling and babbling. He had no issues whatsoever, and then, after his

MMR shot, slowly the smiles and the eye contact faded. The babbling stopped. There was a wall between him and us.

At first, we joked. "He takes being a baby *very* seriously."

When he was three, he would take blades of grass, lay them on the front porch, and make the alphabet. He was really into the letters F and H.

We were thinking: *We have a genius on our hands!* The last thing on our minds was a disability.

Then we got the phone call from the preschool.

Peter was sensitive to loud sounds. If another child cried or screamed, he would go for their faces. That's what happened. He had a fingernail that we hadn't rounded off. There was blood. It wasn't good. Peter was kicked out of school.

There was something in my soul that said, "They're right. Something is wrong with Peter."

He lined things up. He spun in circles.

In many ways his younger brother, Tommy, became the older brother. Tommy began to speak for Peter in a beauti-ful, beautiful way. Even though Peter would get violent and want kids to get away from him, he would let Tommy stay in his face and always bring him toys. It was so lovely.

I would put on movies for the kids, and I'd look for hope on the Internet. I'd Google "social and emotional delays" and always arrived at the A-word, autism. It's heartbreaking to see your child, who is your heart and soul, reduced to these little behaviors. You start to ask, "Is this blade-of-grass thing my child or autism?" I felt like I didn't know Peter any more.

Years before, I had received a Christmas card from a friend I had lost touch with. It said that her son was diagnosed with autism, and gave an update of how they were trying a special diet. I thought she was so out there. Autism is autism.

So, I called my friend on the phone and told her about the preschool. I described his behavior and I asked about the diet, which she told me had cleaned up a lot of her son's behaviors.

I was standing up talking on the phone and I felt my sense of gravity leave, and I just went on my knees. She said, "Well, he really craved milk."

Before that I wouldn't have thought anything of it. We're good American parents. We give our kids milk. But Peter was putting away a lot of milk, obsessively so. Rubbing the refrigerator. Always "milk, milk, milk."

The thought is that some kids have leaky guts. Casein is a protein in milk that if it gets in the blood, it acts like morphine. If that happens, the kids kind of act like they are stoned.

It was so simple to try, so we tried it.

The next ten days were staggering. We saw our son go through the equivalent of a heroin withdrawal. He got the shakes, slept all day, and woke up with raccoon circles under his eyes. It would have frightened us to death, but language, original language came in like gangbusters at the same time. Five-to-twelve-word sentences. Stuff we couldn't believe.

We watched our son come back to us. It's almost like we were meeting him for the first time. He was saying, "I love you." There were all of these Hallmark card moments happening ten times per day.

The first little tiny thing we tried was a jackpot. We were like, "What else ya got?"

I made an appointment with a very well-respected pediatric allergist. I shared this whole story with him. At this point we had no clue we were part of some counter-culture movement.

He looked at me and said, "I believe that you believe that happened, but it didn't happen."

———

The company line of mainstream medicine says that what happens in digestion can't affect our brains whatsoever.

They don't believe it.

My husband had been through medical school. He was so proud of that. But this one aspect—our child's health— was not supported by anything he was taught.

Doctors are taught to medicate, not to fix with nutrition.

We know there are people out there who don't believe in the diets or the shots. We have so much compassion and solidarity and deep feelings for folks who are walking this road. But we can't even begin to have a conversation with many of them because they don't believe in the shot's thing. This story is not their story.

Our reality was very different.

There's a lot of discussion about accepting, about aides, and wills, and we just can't be a part of that. We ran and said, "Autism? Make it go the hell away."

Biomedical intervention believes that autism is reversible. We believe that all people on the spectrum can improve by trying some of these things and some will recover.

We are not unique. There are so many stories of families, but we are "anecdotal evidence."

With autism, you become the doctor. You become the specialist in your child. But a lot of people can't make that shift. People are so willing to turn over the power to the therapists, the experts, and the doctors. That voice inside of you has to be the guide.

The children are leading us. There is something that this whole epidemic is telling us as parents and as a nation.

We believe there is this multi-faceted chemical-induced thing that is happening and then something sets it over the edge. Vaccinations, food, pesticides, exposure to heavy metals, all of these things can add up to autism.

We tried everything: stem cells in Ecuador, heavy metal detox, homeopathy, even a shaman. We dove in deep and maintained this idea of never arriving, and that we would just keep looking, hoping, and believing. And we constantly saw progress.

The real traditional piece that we did was the ABA. It put us in charge. It taught us how to maneuver him. How to control his will; his strong will that controlled our lives.

Peter started first grade with a full-time aide in a mainstream classroom, by third grade he had been accepted into a program for students with high abilities.

Things were going great, and that's when the unthinkable happened.

Tommy, almost three, our baby boy, Peter's number one therapist, died unexpectedly.

He just had a cold, went to sleep, and never woke up. We

have no idea what happened. One day he was here and one day he was gone.

It was during that really dark period when we started to see the value of autism. You try to come out of your own dark reality and think: *How can I guide my son who has lost his brother? How is this going to affect his psyche?"*

But Peter was fine. He had his movies, his Lego's. He was never that bonded with Tommy because he was kind of removed, getting better, but removed. They did interact. They would throw rocks in the creek together on the farm, but it was sort of one-way.

That was an intellectual and emotional shift to say there was value in autism. That it was protecting him from this horrible loss. He was going to be okay.

The autism journey brought my husband and me together. We began to find a way of coping, and since coping was already an integral part of our relationship, autism prepared us for the grief. Coping and healing were woven into our fabric already.

———

The love that we've felt in the Muncie community is overwhelming. Our community is now so much at the theatre.

There was a guest director from Ball State directing *Joseph* at the Civic Theatre. Peter was eight. He got in the show even though there were only a few spots in the children's choir. My husband got in, and I was cast as Potiphar's wife.

So, we're all in *Joseph*. Life was good. Life was getting better. We were hopeful.

We were trying on our costumes for the first time, and we were all having fun. I was practicing my dance when I turned around and the kid who was playing Joseph had just put on his coat for the first time. He was preening and swirling and the coat was flying around.

The coat was made of my circus curtains from the farmhouse, which I forgot I had donated.

I felt punched in the gut, and I couldn't breathe. Here was this fabric that represented such tragedy. And there it was transformed into this beautiful, beautiful thing that was also part of our new story and part of our transformation. It was just amazing.

Every night through the rehearsals and the performance, I felt like everyone was where they were supposed to be. It was so magical.

Our autism journey gave us a belief in healing, and then the grand challenge became can we heal from the loss of Tommy? But that's sort of what we do. We believe in healing.

We can heal. We can be transformed. The more we open up ourselves to this idea of healing, the truer it becomes.

There's no part of the words autism or death that isn't painful.

It's okay if you cry. It's good. It's part of it. It's part of the sadness and the sweetness. It's all tied together.

The tears honor the journey.

9

COMPUTER BRAIN (2021)

KATHRYN DAVIS'S STORY AS TOLD TO CHRISTINE
RHINE

I love my kids so much. I tell everyone about them. Both Michael and Joseph have an autism diagnosis, but they are so different. It's not possible to tell someone, "Go here, and this will work for you," because what works for me may not work for you. Each child is so different.

Michael is adopted from the Philippines. We'd been asked to host him while he had an operation here in Fort Wayne, but as soon as he got off the plane, we knew we would never send him back. He was born with a hole in his skull, and his doctors had simply given up hope after trying many times to stitch him back together. He's essentially had five lobotomies. He'll never be able to live alone, but he and Joseph are inseparable, and I think eventually they will be able to make it by helping each other. Their sister, Madison, is adopted from China, and she is what I call neurotypical. People say, "Oh, is she normal?" and I say, "No, none of us are normal. She is neurotypical." The kids are all very close, and I know if I cannot always care for them, they will stick together. I have a trust and guardianship already in place for them.

We'd only had Michael and Madison for a short time—they are only six months apart in age—when the family who had been going to adopt Joseph decided they couldn't take him. They'd been told his vocal cords were paralyzed, and he'd never be able to speak. Today Joseph speaks. He's a savant artist, one in one-hundred thousand people are savant artists. He's a man of few words, but he speaks volumes through his art. He can look at a building and draw it—to the brick—from memory. He draws ships, down to the bolt. It's amazing.

We knew something was up with him from the moment he arrived. From the airport, we took him to Cracker Barrel, and at two or two-and-a-half-years-old (we don't know his exact age) he repeatedly did that tabletop puzzle where you move the tees around a pyramid. Who does that? What baby can do that?

Michael has an eidetic memory for the things that interest him. He knows everything about Greek mythology, Roman mythology.

The boys both graduated from high school. Michael was in a program that included working at a job in the community. He works at a church, and they love him there. They were happy to let him continue working after graduation, so he works three days a week. He has a clipboard, and he's very serious about getting all the trash cans emptied. He loves that job!

Joseph helps me pack Michael's lunch. Joseph is also my landscaper and my pool boy.

My husband and I fell into that percentage of special needs families that divorce. When we were together, we established a foundation that brought one-hundred-and-one children to the United States for adoption. I'm a single mother now. I don't let anything slow me down. In ten years, I earned a bachelor's degree, two masters', and a PhD. Sometimes I took the kids into the computer lab with me, armed with Game Boys and snacks, and . . . you know what? They always behaved. I am a professor and department chair at Ivy Tech now. I help train social workers and counselors who will work with special needs children and their families. My boys keep me young. They teach me so many things that I teach my students. I bring them to class sometimes.

It dawned on me one day that I would never have an empty nest. It's okay. They make me laugh every day. They say the funniest things. I have no regrets. Sometimes you have to look at where life has led you, the good things you have, not what you don't have.

My advice is to meet your child in their world rather than trying to drag him into our world. I promise, you will find his abilities there. It's cute. It's funny. It's okay to be different.

Once a little girl asked Michael what was wrong with him. He said, "I have a special computer in my brain. It's called autism. What's wrong with you?" I tried not to laugh. It's okay to embrace our differences.

None of us are normal. Besides, sometimes roller coasters can be fun.

10

JOURNEYING FROM DISBELIEF TO ACCEPTANCE (2013)

ANNIE TIMMERMAN'S STORY AS TOLD TO BETH MESSNER

Thinking about a time when...
I wasn't filled with anxiety...
I didn't routinely compare my son to other children his age...
I used to take photos for family scrapbooks...
I wasn't constantly looking for "red flags"...
we were a carefree family.
Thinking about how...
he enjoys watching Peppa Pig on TV...
he laughs when his father swings him through the air...
he loves to make animal sounds...
he likes to draw with sidewalk chalk...
he wraps his hands in my hair when we cuddle...
I'm thinking about my son Griffin Noah, a sweet, quiet, two-year-old who has autism.

———

Mine was the proverbial small town "growing up." Everybody knew everybody in my rural community. I've known my husband since we were kids. We were high school sweethearts—our first date was at a homecoming dance. Eleven years later, we married. We had two children, one who shares his middle name with his great-great-great-grandfather. We had planned a wonderful life for our family. Then we received the news...

That news was broken to me during Griffin's fifteen-month wellness visit with his pediatrician. While my husband and I noticed that his development was somewhat delayed, we weren't horribly concerned. Sure, he was developing slowly, but he would catch up to his peers...

The completed development questionnaire in the pediatrician's hands suggested a different story. Griffin's inability to engage in pretend play, his ritualistic behaviors, difficulties communicating, and problems connecting with others —all of these, we learned, were signs of autism.

Disbelief. Fear. Denial. Anger. Uncertainty. Guilt. It's amazing the places that your heart and head can go when grappling with such news.

We were overwhelmed. We didn't know anything about autism, didn't know anyone whose children had autism.

As we desperately trolled the internet for information, our understanding increased, but so did our fears. We imagined the worst. Our hopes for Griffin's future were dashed. We only shared the news with a few people, not sure whether the doctor was correct, not willing to believe that his pronouncement could be true. We kept scrutinizing Griffin's behaviors and comparing them to the list of "red flags," asking ourselves, "Is this autism or is this being a two-year-old?"

We held out hope when symptoms weren't obvious or appeared mild. When asked, a few family members and friends admitted that they had concerns about Griffin that they hadn't expressed to us prior to the doctor's visit. I felt guilty. They saw problems that I felt I, as Griffin's mother, *should* have seen. But I didn't. I stopped asking because I had a really hard time handling it.

During this time, I also experienced an overwhelming desire to do something to try to "fix" Griffin's problems. We continued our relentless search for information and advice, made appointments with other physicians to examine Griffin, arranged for him to receive therapy, even put our family on a gluten- and casein-free diet. We felt an incredible need to exert some degree of control over our situation.

Now I think I've reached a level of acceptance.

My son has autism.

In some ways, my days are not terribly unlike those experienced by other mothers: dropping the kids off at the childcare center, going to the gym, taking family bike rides, spending quiet time with my husband, sitting down to family dinners. But always the specter of autism haunts us . .
.

Three times a week, a therapist visits our home to work with Griffin. The parks we visit must be fenced so he doesn't run off. We put a piece of bright tape across the end of our driveway to signal Griffin to stop so he won't run into the street. Public excursions make me anxious because people might notice Griffin is different and judge him for it.

Perhaps our most heart-breaking challenge? Helping our four-year-old daughter understand why her little brother is not like other two-year-olds. I choke up when she says, "I don't know what's wrong with Griffy, but I still love him."

I'm also grateful. I'm grateful that Griffin's autism is mild and that he is making progress in his therapy sessions. As difficult as it is to adjust to an autistic child, our family does not face the same challenges as those whose children have more severe disabilities. While Griffin has difficulty communicating with others and likes to do things certain ways, he doesn't get *stuck* performing behaviors, unable to break free. And, we can definitely see improvements in his ability to socialize and to adapt to unfamiliar environments.

Our family and friends have been very supportive throughout this process. For this, I also am grateful. Our parents spend time caring for both children and help Griffin learn to interact and feel comfortable in unfamiliar situations. Friends regularly ask about him and listen to my stories and concerns. I've also developed an informal network with other mothers who have children with autism. This is perhaps the most valuable therapy for me. These are the people who *really* know what it's like. They understand what I am feeling and thinking, the challenges I face, because they have been there themselves.

As the mother of a child with autism, I'm definitely in a better place now, even though I still have many things to learn and challenges to face. Now, I can see down the road and be more optimistic. Ten years from now, I hope to see Griffin in school, interacting with his peers, and learning. I hope he'll be in a regular classroom instead of attending special education classes. Most of all, I hope that Griffin understands his disorder and is okay with it.

11

CAMERON'S JOURNEY (2021)

ANGIE, ANDY AND CAMERON HOESMAN'S STORY AS TOLD TO JULES CARTER

W hen I first laid eyes on Cameron, I knew. I didn't know what I "knew," but I knew...

He was in preschool when we got the diagnosis.

It was his preschool teacher from Head Start who told us we would need to find an inclusive classroom.

I knew nothing about where to go for help. This was sixteen years ago and people in our situation were few and far between.

The first person we found laid a foundation of exploration to find different services to help our son. A co-worker recommended a coffee date with Belinda Hughes to help me navigate what to do. She was incredible and started helping us find programs for Cameron.

On a whim, we taught Cameron a few words in sign language. He still uses them today. They are helpful when he is excited and can't access his words fast enough or really wants our attention.

The more people we encountered the more wonderful programs we found.

Yorktown schools were great. Every IEP meeting brought us a new person to help Cameron discover something new.

Judy Scott, from the resource room, started with Cameron in elementary school, and coincidentally moved to middle and high school as Cameron did. She has been pivotal in Cameron's growth. She has a special ability to light him up and get him to work at something.

We found a pediatric rehab group that specializes in improving how the body responds to different senses. In Cameron's journey, this is where his biggest struggle was. After five years of rehab, Cameron was visibly more comfortable and in control of his body.

His ability to focus and his awareness of his surroundings is better than we ever hoped for.

As Cameron grew up, we found many great groups to give him a safe space to socialize.

When we found the Prism project at Ball State University, Cameron went from not participating and standing on the periphery to being up on stage.

In 2019, Cameron was in a two-person show with Muncie Civic's Barrier-Free Theatre program (a drama therapy model to empower adults with intellectual/developmental disabilities). He starred in a skit written just for them. It was like he was meant to be on the stage! It was and is one of the best things for him. His growth has been remarkable.

So many of the people who've helped Cameron are still in our lives, including Belinda. Since then, Belinda started an ABA clinic, Behavior Associates of Indiana (BAI). As he gets older, Cameron looks forward to BAI's local, social group.

Family time is a cornerstone of our lives together. We play games and have fun conversations. Included in our family time is grocery shopping. Cameron *loves* to grocery shop and the whole grocery experience! He loves to gather carts in the parking lot before and after we go in. He has a list and we challenge him to find everything without our assistance. He does amazingly well. It gives him the opportunity to engage with cashiers and other employees as needed.

Cameron finished his education in May of 2022.

I was afraid when we started this journey that we wouldn't find what he needed, but we have found so many services that address his needs and the support of a community that has helped us get there.

We have gone from not knowing what Cameron's life will look like, to Cameron having a path forward.

12

AWESTRUCK (2021)

LOGAN CARTER'S STORY ABOUT MEETING CAMERON HOESMAN

When my mom told me about the interview, I kept an open mind and readied myself for anything. We met with the family at my mom's office to ask them a few questions and talk. They brought their 20-year-old son, Cameron, along for the journey as well. My job was simple: Sit and listen with the audio recorder in my hand. I didn't expect it to be too much of a big deal. Oh boy was I wrong.

I didn't gather too much from the actual conversation, but I kept an eye on Cameron. While my mom was talking with his parents, he kept listening to music. No earbuds, no headphones, nothing. He just kept it at a low volume and held it to his ear. I almost immediately recognized the music: *movie soundtracks*. Not like from *John Wick* or *Chappie*. But from kid's movies. I'm talking about *Cars, The Incredibles, How to Train Your Dragon*. That gave me a lot about Cameron's thought process. On the outside, he was a teen, around my age. But on the inside, he was a kid, probably around seven.

Then the real kicker came. Around fifty or so minutes into the interview, we heard a train horn. My mom's office is right next to a set of train tracks, so it wasn't uncommon for trains to pass. However, when the horn sounded, Cameron perked up. He paused the music and asked if that was a train we just heard. When they answered yes, he asked if he could go see it. So, my mom asked me to escort him outside so he could watch it pass.

When he saw the train, his eyes lit up like a Christmas tree. He made claims like "That's so cool!" and "I'm so happy!" And these quotes were genuine joy coming from this guy. Watching Cameron be awestruck by a train reminded me of the things in my childhood that I was awestruck by. That's when it dawned on me how significant his condition was. He's never going to be able to live on his own. He's always going to have to have someone as his "guardian."

Cameron isn't the only one with this condition. There are tens of thousands, possibly millions, of kids and teens like him that live like he does. They need all the support they can get. And that's where we come in. I'm not talking like donating money or anything (although you can totally donate to autism awareness groups if you want). I'm talking about donating time. Being there for these people so they don't feel alone. And by helping these people, they give back to us. They remind us of the graces that are the small things from our childhood. For me, it was watching trains and listening to movie soundtracks. So, by helping kids and

teens with autism, it doesn't just help them, but it helps us
as well.

13

JOURNALING (2013)

REBECCA TYLER'S STORY AS TOLD TO CHERYL WILLIAMSON

I decided that in spite of what the doctors believed, I would focus on something I could control—his diet.

I became obsessed with keeping track of thirty-two-month-old Luke's daily food intake, his bowel movements, his accomplishments, his regressions. I became a machine when it came to journaling. I was convinced that diet was playing a significant role in keeping him from progressing at the pace of others his age.

At our first visit with the doctor at Riley, we were told that what we thought were milestones appropriate for his age, were in fact nothing; that Luke was behind others who were nearly three years old.

Immediate guilt set in.

At that point, I was a stay-at-home mother of two boys. My younger son was extremely colicky, so I wasn't able to spend much time interacting with Luke when Jake needed my attention. I blamed myself for this lack of interaction; fortunately, the doctor assured me that Luke's diagnosis was not my fault. But how could I have not seen the signs? What I thought was his quirkiness was, in fact, behaviors that placed him on the spectrum.

I clearly remember the doctor arguing with me about Luke's early achievements. I simply thought that Luke was a bit laid back, like his father. I also told myself that he is a boy; that he is the oldest, so his language would eventually come. Of course, I had no benchmarks with which to compare him. Because I had never been around other toddlers, I wasn't looking for anything to be wrong.

My obsession with journaling was paying off. As I journaled, I began to realize that Luke was losing and gaining language. And then Jake, his younger sibling, began talking and was soon surpassing Luke's speech. At this point, I knew I had to do something constructive to help out Luke.

I began reading everything I could get a hold of that dealt with autism. Too often what I was reading hit too close to home and reinforced the doctor's diagnosis. I spent a lot of time crying. I became depressed. Keeping the journal was something constructive I could focus on. And because I am not a very patient person, and because the changes in Luke's behavior were often gradual, keeping the journal allowed me to look back and see that he had indeed made improvements.

I was afraid that maybe his diet was giving him headaches or somehow preventing him from developing his language. I wanted to be sure he had every opportunity to be successful. The doctors and the therapists aren't going to argue for a change of diet because controlling diet is not a money maker for them. They were pushing the different therapies: speech and occupational. Yes, the therapies are beneficial, but I firmly believe that the diet was necessary. After all, how can Luke be receptive to learning, if he doesn't feel well?

While the docs and therapists might not be getting rich from a selective diet, the natural food stores surely were. Because I had quit my job to devote myself to raising our two boys, we were at half of our income, and I was implementing a diet that was terribly expensive. A single loaf of specialized bread cost around $6; a half-gallon of ice cream was close to $8. Not only did I change Luke's diet, but I also added supplements and probiotics. Again, not cheap. Luckily, my mother was willing to help us out with purchasing his special diet.

I wrote down every morsel of food, every sip of a beverage that passed his lips. At the same time, I kept track of any milestones or any significant setbacks he was experiencing with the new diet. Often, he would experience withdrawal symptoms when certain foods were removed. He had been very selective about his diet. He would only eat graham crackers, apples, chicken nuggets, peanut butter and jelly, orange juice, and 2% milk. But when I replaced those items, that's when I noticed the withdrawal symptoms. The calm, quiet child became a Tasmanian devil. These trigger items usually contained gluten. "Must be gluten free" became my new mantra as I furiously journaled each and every day.

The process of changing his diet was a gradual one. I had to remove foods one at a time and then add changes. For example, after the 2% milk was removed, I waited a little while and then introduced rice milk. And of course, I kept meticulous track of the changes in diet and his behaviors. I have three years' worth of the food/behavior journals. Someday I hope to find the time to type out the journals to keep as a record of this time.

All the time I was controlling Luke's diet, I was feeding our younger son regular foods. While the food/activity journal validated Luke's need for a specialized diet, I decided to stop the diet when Luke was entering school; when I knew for certain that he could communicate sufficiently with others. I wanted him to be able to blend in with his peers.

The journaling paid off, as did the constant help from therapists, teachers, friends, and family. We began to see some improvements. We've come a long way from wishing he could just verbalize what he wants, to listening to him belt out all the words to a Maroon 5 song. From wondering how to get him to hold the pencil correctly, to finding his name on the wall and engraved into the furniture; his brother got the blame for that!

And while a combination of therapies and a change of diet helped Luke find his language, I firmly believe that Jake, his younger brother and scapegoat, now is his best therapy.

14

HOME PLATE (2013)

DENNIS LEE TYLER'S STORY AS TOLD TO CHERYL WILLIAMSON

I've come a long way in overcoming my fears from that first moment of Luke's diagnosis when I thought he would never be able to fully participate in organized sports and feel a part of a team; when I thought he would not ever speak. While he is still not mindful of his own space, he is able to understand direction from his coach, and he is able to communicate.

The predictions of the doctor at Riley were dire. He had a four in seven chance of having mental retardation. He likely wouldn't speak beyond what he was at that time, which was not at all. I wanted to jump across the table, to shake the doctor, to tell him he was wrong. "My son can't be autistic! How will he ever be able to play T-ball or run track or do any activity where he must take direction and communicate?"

I refused to believe the doctor. After all, I was at Riley in the first place *only* because my father urged me to have my son tested for his lack of speech.

Prior to Luke's birth, my father, a State Representative, was a member of the Statehouse Autism Committee. He was knowledgeable about the symptoms and what to look for. He didn't come right out and say to me, "Son, I believe Luke is autistic." Instead, because Luke was completely non-verbal at the time, Dad urged us to have his speech tested. We called Riley to get an appointment for the testing, and it was set up for six months from the day of our call. Six months! We couldn't believe it. But luckily, Dad pulled some strings and got us in within two weeks. Without his intercession, we would have lost an entire six months of therapies.

At that first diagnostic appointment, the doctor asked us the question, "What do you think Luke should be doing at this stage of his life?" When we stated what we believed he had accomplished, the doctor assured us that Luke was not exhibiting behavior typical of a three-year old. We left that appointment and cried; I cried tears of anger, of frustration. However, I decided that we were fortunate. We had a diagnosis; one that wasn't as dire as I had first thought it could be. My son wasn't wearing braces; he wasn't going to be a teenager wearing diapers.

We had a label we could work with.

That label, however, could be a double-edged sword. Yes, he was now labeled as autistic, but that label could work to his advantage by offering him help, as needed. I used to stress about thinking of what would happen to Luke if something happened to my wife Becca or me. I still stress on occasion, but I now firmly believe he will be fine. He will have enough resources and enough help to see him through any situation.

Another issue Luke has to overcome is that he is just too darn cute. Because he is so cute, people have a tendency to help him, which quite quickly turns into enabling him. They often won't let him do for himself. He isn't allowed to work through his quirks without others coming to his aid. This can be a hindrance to progression.

Even though he is quirky, Luke is wicked smart. He can talk to you about any type of shark that exists. Ask him about dinosaurs and he can talk about them in detail. If he is interested in a subject, he embraces it whole-heartedly.

When he began kindergarten, I had many fears for him. Would he make friends? Would he be able to play with the other children? Would he be picked on? Would he even know it if he *was* being picked on? The list of the fears I had for him goes on and on. His second day of school, I left work early so I could stop in at the school to see how he was doing. As soon as his teacher saw me, she said, "He's going to be just fine." I immediately burst into tears! Many of those fears on my list now have been deleted.

Last summer, we had a defining moment in his progress, or maybe I should say in my progress. While participating on a T-ball team, Luke, the son who I feared would never play sports, hit the ball and ran the bases. As he crossed home plate, he looked up at us in the stands and gave us a thumb's up. I knew right then and there that while we might not always experience positives, that at that particular moment in time, Luke was experiencing a feeling of happiness and of gratitude and of a sense of belonging. And I was too.

My son will be just fine.

15

CASPER (2021)

DEBBIE DUBOIS' STORY AS TOLD TO DAROLYN "LYN" JONES

"Casper," he whispered to me in a hushed, anxious tone. "Casper," he repeated, louder and with more urgency.

"Grandma will be right back to play with you, I promise! You play my turn this time, okay?"

"C'mon, Joel, let's head to the kitchen so you can tell me again about the computer you are working on. And thank you for being patient, buddy."

Casper was the friendly ghost, a lovable ghost that sometimes still shows up on the TV Land Channel. But he was also a very lonely ghost. He didn't fit in with other ghosts because he wasn't interested in scaring people, so he left and wondered the world trying to find humans who weren't scared of him. He wanted friends, to be included, and to be a living child again—to be typical. He found a family, a mother with two children who became his fast friends, a family who accepted him.

When my ninety-eight-year-old father-in-law was living with us, Joel walked up to me and said, "Mom, I feel invisible." Casper.

My heart sank. Caretaking my father-in-law and my son was challenging. Taking care of Joel was also challenging, rewarding yes, but still challenging. So, I said, "Okay, Joel, let's come up with a code word so when you need a hug or my attention, I can stop and give that to you." He looked down at me (he's 6 foot 2, so he has to look down to look in my eyes, something he doesn't do often) and said in a hushed tone, "Casper."

When I think about that lonely, invisible ghost wanting to be included, seen, heard, I have to wonder if that's why he chose this word. I don't know, but what I do know is that he still uses it. Most folks who hear it, don't get it and that's okay. It's our secret mother/son language. We know what it means.

I'm the mother of two girls in their 30s, one with two children of her own, so I am also a grandmother. And I'm the mother of a nineteen-year-old son, Joel. Joel wasn't only an "oops" baby, but he is also my only boy and my only child who has autism. Like Casper, Joel is high functioning, but doesn't fit in as well, even with other kids who have autism. He struggles to find acceptance.

Here's what I want you know about my son: he's been failed, even rejected over and over by public and parochial schools. Listen to some of the hurtful and ignorant excuses I have heard over the years:

"He's just spoiled; there's nothing wrong with him."

"He'll never read."

"We can't accept your child at our school because academically, he couldn't survive."

I opted to home school him because I don't see my son's gifts as a deficit. My mantra is "If something isn't working, then change it." And so, I did.

I remember when we received his first diagnosis, Asperger's. And I remember thinking, *Thank God, it's not autism.* But in what was one of many misdiagnoses and mistakes made by the medical community, it turned out that he did have autism.

Joel has anxiety and a heightened fear of doctors. Once put under anesthesia for a routine procedure, he didn't receive enough and remembered and felt too much. You take that trauma and marry it with autism and it's tricky.

Joel LOVES computers and all things Bill Gates. He can take apart and put back together any PC computer system with an XP platform. He knows the history, make, model, and year of every computer and system Gates developed. He even dressed up like Gates for Halloween. I mean, what kid does that? Mine does. My Joel. My funny boy who tells jokes like: "What does the tornado say to the twister? Let's go for a spin!"

Joel loves the Prism project in Muncie. He even emceed the event, telling his jokes. He was a hit! I wish this kind of programming happened all year. Because it's one of those few places he can go and feel included, and where I can see what he really can do. It's a space where we both feel hope.

When your life becomes about advocating, taking your son to therapy appointments, to social groups, and constantly worrying about your son's future, your ability to socialize is tough. Family is so much more supportive now than they used to be. They finally are starting to see it and get it. But I have had to leave my job to take care of him; old friends don't, or rarely, call on me anymore. Kids his age are going to college, have girlfriends, jobs. He wants what they have, but can't access it. I would like to have typical friendships too, but it's not accessible to me anymore either.

But I have found a wonderful support system with another mother of a son with autism in Ohio. We connected years ago and can call each other, drop everything to be there for one another. It's a special relationship. Like my son and I, she and I share a special language. Mothers get it.

Sometimes a total stranger does, too. I remember once taking Joel to the Hobby Lobby to grab some supplies, and he was whining and becoming increasingly loud and agitated and he's again, tall—a big kid. There were stares. I kept him on my arm and kept talking with him. A woman behind me in line came up to my opposite side and said, "I work with kids like your son. Mom, you're doing a great job." This total stranger gets what I'm going through. I got in my car and cried.

That one moment was special because when we are out, we are usually confronted with ugly, misunderstood stares. I remember when our neighbors called the cops because they thought my son was threatening my husband. My husband had taken him outside for a walk after he was particularly agitated because it's an activity that calms him down. But his outbursts and size were interpreted as a threat.

I do a lot of talking about my son. I worry that because

he looks typical, he will be judged or hurt. What I wish people knew is that I love my son fiercely and I want him to be independent, included, and loved. I want what any mother would want for her child.

And most importantly, I want more people to get it.

A PERSONAL STORY ABOUT A PERSONAL COMPUTER (2021)

JOEL DUBOIS' STORY AS TOLD TO DAROLYN "LYN" JONES

A binary system is a two base number system made up of only two numbers or digits: 0 and 1. Off or On. The binary system was created by German mathematician Gottfried Wilhelm Leibniz. Leibniz was not just a mathematician, but also a philosopher with deep convictions about religion, philosophy, and morality. According to every account I came across about his life, he was described as a passionate and positive person who tried to make sense of the world through multiple lenses, mathematics being what he was most known for. Oxford Bibliographies calls Leibniz, a universal genius (para. 1). Without Leibniz's passion and calling, we wouldn't have the computer, a device that all of us use and rely upon for even the most basic access to information and services.

According to Computer Hope (2021), computers use the binary system because the 0 and 1 system can quickly detect that the computer is in the false (off) or true (on) position. And having only those two states means the distance apart makes the computer less susceptible to electrical interference (paras. 1-3).

Joel DuBois and Gottfried Leibniz have much in common. They both love the binary system and they both believe passionately in how simplistic, yet beautiful the computing system has been in creating a technology process that has changed the trajectory of the world *and* they both believe passionately in preserving that system.

When anxiety started to impact Joel's autism and life, he took medications, he saw doctors, he learned how to tell when the anxiety was coming on so he could employ strategies to get it under control before it controlled him. And during that long year of battling his anxiety, someone brought him an old personal computer (PC), and he fixed it. Thus began his passion and love for all things related to the PC.

According to Geeks on Site (2018), computers include the following components:

- CPU: A Central Processing Unit that handles operations and functions;
- RAM: Random Access Memory where all data is stored so the CPU can access and process;
- HDD: Hard Disk Drive where all of our photos, apps, docs are kept;
- Motherboard which is the home for all other components which allows them to each communicate with each other. No motherboard; no computer;
- Video and Sound Cards: This component allows

us to hear and see what the computer is
processing; and a
- Network adapter: How we connect to the
Internet and all of that wonderful information!
(para. 3.)

Joel's central unit processes operations and functions
through his unique and brilliant lens of autism. He recalls
months, years, and key events like a computer. His memory
is much like a hard disk drive because Joel can tell you
about every PC he has used, was given, or that he
purchased, took apart, and put back together. And with
serious sadness, he talks of the PCs he lost and couldn't
save.

His motherboard is Debbie DuBois. His mother is his
strongest advocate and champion. The first time I met
Debbie, she had organized notes in hand, ready to tell me
the stories of every medical, educational, and family
members she had to either battle against to get Joel the
services he needed to flourish or that championed along-
side her. Joel's network is much like how a computer
connects, a series of wires, fibers, and links that talk to
each other to support the process. Joel connects to the
world through his parents, his family, his friends, his
work, but most profoundly through his love of all
things PC.

A tinkerer, like his dad, Joel can take a PC completely
apart and put it back together. The PC might have been
broken to begin with, and it might not have been. It doesn't
matter. That wonder of seeing all of those mesmerizing
parts strewn out on his bed while he pieces them back

together to run Windows again are a critical connection and contribution to the world for Joel.

Joel's room is wrapped in layered shelving that hold and situate his vast PC collection. He ensures they have equal space so if running, they don't overheat. Friends and families or folks who just know Joel give him their old PC computers, working or not. His deal with his mom is that when the shelves and floors below are full, if a new one comes in, one has to be donated out. His current collection houses 30 PCs.

Joel told me about his life through his PCs and the events those PCs experienced. The PC is personified as Joel talks. For Joel, these machines are living and breathing.

I remember in 2003, my dad opened up an old Window's PC that belonged to my uncle. It was a Pentium 2 or 3, had floppy disks. It was so cool.

I remember playing Sesame Street and Peter Rabbit games on my dad's Pentium 3 Dell computer.

I remember being in the first computer lab in my old school in 2002, the room full of Windows XP 98 computers.

As Joel started talking with me about his passion for all things PC, his "remembers" became stories.

In 2014, my dad brought home an old Dell computer. We were outside and he said, "Go look behind that fence. There is something out there you would like. I don't know if it will work, but we can try it out." It was an old PC. We cleaned it out, then plugged it in, and it made this noise (fan whirring noise). It fired up! Windows XP Home edition Service Pack 2, a Pentium 4, a black and beautiful Dell.

When it couldn't boot up anymore, I decided to work on it. I had pieces scattered everywhere. My mom came into my room, looked around, and just closed the door. I got it working again. It was trial and error. Sometime in 2015, when that black Dell was on its final straws, I tried to get it to work. I couldn't. It was over. I was sad it was over. But I still have that hard drive.

My brother had this old HP computer from 2002, and it ran an actual Windows Whistler Windows Titan 3. It was a gray HP. I liked the gray vintage look of it. I loved the sound it made when it fired up because it was really loud. I loved the sound. In 2017 I did some diagnostics on it, but I touched the cord on the hard drive, and it made this sad noise and shut down. That was very last time it worked. The HP PC works, but the hard drive doesn't.

Last year we found a new hard drive for it, and I'm going to use it as donor hard drive. Just like a donor organ, there is a 50/50 chance it will work.

In 2011, my grandpa had a very old PC, a Gateway computer with a Pentium 4. I don't know what happened to it, but I remember it and I'm still looking for that very model. It was loud and had a green light fan that was different from anything else.

I once had a Dell that overheated. That Dell fought for its life. We sprayed it with a fire extinguisher and that Dell kept fighting through the fire, but it died.

When I asked Joel if he could change anything about the PC machine he loves, knows, and works on, he became very serious. Joel expressed that he is upset about the social media movement of people smashing PCs and taking videos of it and posting it to the Internet, and he became visibly and audibly agitated when discussing this disturbing new trend.

When I come across one of those videos— which sometimes pop up when I am looking things up online— it makes me sick.

You are smashing PC history. These machines are fully functional. Just wipe the hard drive. Ask for help if you don't know how to do it. These machines can still work and be used and be saved. Don't tear them apart, smash them, or throw them away —I'll take them.

And viruses. Virus are the PC's enemy. Joel wishes he could come up with a way to run any game or Windows program without fear of a virus. And he hopes that he or someone can come up with a way to send back that virus meant to kill a PC back to the virus creator and sender.

I reminded Joel that we were talking to him because this was to be a story about how he faces autism. And was there anything else he wanted to share about how he faces autism. He turned his attention to others with autism instead. His advice to others who are facing autism is this:

Don't let people push you around. I am smart. Don't let people tell you are stupid—I'm not.

There are mean people out there. But I'm cheering you on and supporting you.

Different isn't always bad.

Different can be good.

Binary. (11, October 2021). Computer hope. https://www. computerhope.com/jargon/b/binary.htm

Geeks on Site. (13, August 2018). How does a computer work. https://geeksonsite.com/blog/how-does-a-computer-work/

Strickland, L. (2021). Gottfried Willhelm Leibniz. Oxford Bibliographies. https://www.oxfordbibliographies.com/view/document/obo-9780195399301/obo-9780195399301-0359.xml

17

BLUE DRAGON AVATAR: BRIAN'S POEM (2013)

BRIAN WHITE'S STORY AS TOLD TO MICHAEL BROCKLEY

I n the fourth grade, I asked my mom why I had a bad brain. She promised me I'd always be wonderful. I'd repeated second grade. Two years later, I spent too much time jumping on the trampoline in the sensory room. I never liked to read. Disliked math and AP history. But graduated from Southside with honors. I suffered death threats as a senior. Bullies are worthless scumbags.

I play Mortal Kombat and Uncharted as Blue Dragon, the warrior who shoots blue fire from the palms of his hands. I climb skyscrapers to combat the thugs and mercenaries in the adventures I imagine. There are no superpowers in Uncharted. In battle, I fight with my fists. To play Manga and Pokémon, I learned to read and write Japanese.

At Cousin Vinny's, I wash dishes and take pizza orders over the phone. Sometimes, I bake the Deluxes and Veggie Revivals. I take my turn walking the advertisement along McGalliard. I don't have to dress like a lizard. Just work clothes. Khaki pants and shirts without neckties. I answer the questions asked of me. If the answer is yes, I say "yes." I say "no" when the answer is no.

After attending church for all the wrong reasons, I came to Jesus at fourteen. The only book I've ever enjoyed is the Bible. Matthew says, "For if you forgive others when they sin against you, your heavenly Father will also forgive you." I wear robin's egg blue neckties to worship. Taught myself to tie four-in-hand knots. I am learning to forgive.

Sometimes I need days to answer questions my friends can answer with the snap of a finger. The left side of my brain works less than the right side. I want to program video games and work in Japan. My mom said I'd always be wonderful.

18

MY SON, THE PROM KING (2013)

EMMA OSBORN'S STORY AS TOLD TO LISA COMBS

My story is a lot different than parents who have young kids with autism now. See, my kid didn't *have* autism twenty years ago. Oh, he *had* autism. I just couldn't get anyone to *say* he had autism.

It was a different world then and it was a rare diagnosis at the time. I was told over and over that I was just an overly concerned mom. I was just an inexperienced, over-reactive young mom. I just didn't have another child to compare him to. After all, kids develop at different rates, right?

Even his dad thought I was being paranoid.

But a mother knows. I knew.

Of course, I didn't know it was autism. I didn't even know what autism was. I didn't have a word for it, but I knew something was wrong. And I wanted a word for it. I would go to the doctors' appointments and tell them, "My baby won't smile. My baby won't cuddle with me. My baby isn't trying to make sounds. Listen to me! My baby rolls *away* from me!"

But no. I was just a crazy mom. After all, he was hitting a lot of other . . . what do they call them . . . developmental milestones? He walked early. Never even crawled. That's gotta be a positive, right? You look for things—anything—to reassure yourself that your kid is ok. My kid didn't even "bother" crawling. He just skipped right to walking! He could put any puzzle you gave him together. Perfectly. *Perfectly* . . . but upside down.

Then there was the rocking and the head banging.

And I felt like I was banging my head, too. Until one day, at the lab I work at, I was talking to a geneticist about Brian. And she listened. Thank God, finally someone listened. Nobody but a parent who has been there can understand why getting a diagnosis is a good thing. But if you've been there, you know what a relief it is to finally have a name for it. The diagnosis gave Brian a chance to get into a special preschool class. He didn't speak yet, so at school they taught him to use signs and pictures to communicate his needs. It turned out he was actually incredibly smart and perceptive. But at home? We didn't need sign language or pictures. I was so tuned in with him that we didn't even need words.

I remember one night, Brian was upset about something and he was just standing, like he often did, banging his head over and over on the wall. I was exhausted, watching him bang his head over and over. I finally asked him, "Baby, why do you do that? Doesn't that hurt you?" He stopped and looked at me and shook his head "no." Then he went back to banging his head. I got out of my chair and walked to the wall. I stood next to him and, without a word, I started banging my head, too. I hadn't banged it more than a few times when I felt his hand on my arm, pulling me away from the wall. I knelt and looked him in the eye. He shook his head and rubbed my forehead with his little hand. He wanted me to stop so I wouldn't hurt myself. So much for kids with autism not understanding emotions.

Finally, he started to speak, which made some things much easier and some things much harder. Once he could talk, I started to hear how hard life was for him. He came home from school one day and asked me, "Mom, why was I born with a bad brain? Was I bad? Does God hate me?" What could I say to that? I told him, "Maybe you're not the one with a bad brain. Maybe the rest of us are the ones with bad brains."

I never made excuses for my son. I know that the world doesn't give anyone a break. I had my own share of tough times in the world, and I knew that it was going to be even harder for Brian. So, I decided that no one was going to pat my kid on the head, tell me how cute and polite he was, and what a pleasure he was to have in class and then just pass him on to the next teacher. He was going to get everything he needed to meet all the academic expectations of any other child in school; I would see to that.

I had to fight for him to be retained twice in elementary school so he could catch up with the other kids. They told me that he would never be normal no matter how many times he was held back. They told me that I was just in denial. But I felt like I had to make sure Brian had every opportunity to learn. It seemed like everyone wanted to help *me* accept my son's limitations instead of helping *him* to overcome them.

In 1995, Indiana instituted the autism waiver (and I should probably knock wood that it doesn't fall victim to this crappy economy). It wasn't exactly a pile of money, considering all the services Brian needed, but it changed *everything.* Suddenly we weren't alone. It paid for us to hire a consultant to pave the road ahead of us, plus training and support for his teachers. He went from a separate class in a special school to being almost fully included in regular classes by middle school.

And yet all along the way, what did people keep asking me? "Why are you doing this to your son? Why are you putting him through this? Why are you putting the schools through this? Why can't you just accept your son the way he is?" Those questions were answered the day Brian graduated high school, eighth in his class, and was handed his Honors Diploma.

I still worry about him, but not for the same reasons. After all, he has long since put to rest any questions about his academic potential. He is now a sophomore at Ball State, majoring in computer science and minoring in Japanese. Don't get me wrong, he has to work for it. Doing well in school is as important to him as volunteering at church. I know that he will graduate, get a good job, and live a responsible life.

But he still has anxiety and great difficulty understanding social relationships. But it is a myth that kids with autism don't want or need friends. He is *way* more intuitive about emotions and seems to feel everything more intensely than anyone I know. He doesn't bang his head anymore, but I'm sure he often feels like it.

He has such a gentle spirit that people just seem to gravitate to him. It is common for people to come up to us and tell Brian how he is an inspiration to them. But no one calls him to go to the movies. He wants so much to have friends, to date, and to fall in love and get married someday. He even knows how many kids he wants: *two*—a boy and a girl. I keep reminding him that it's not quite that simple to plan.

The dating thing is so hard. He got set up on a date for prom and was so excited, but the girl had some of her own issues and ended up bailing on him at the last minute. No problem, though. Three girls who had come dateless decided they needed him to be their escort, and he had a blast. Especially when he was crowned Prom King later that night!

Back when Brian was little, I resisted putting him on medications because I was always afraid it would change his loving, kind personality or ruin his creativity. But the doctor reminded me that his anxiety and attention issues were holding him back. I'll never forget the doctor saying, "How would you feel if you found out you were denying your son something that could be life-changing for him?"

As I sit in the coffee shop and watch Brian drive off to his job at the pizza place, knowing he will be getting home and hitting the books for hours to be ready for class again tomorrow, I think about how far we have come. I think back to the many times I was asked, "Why are you putting him through this? Why can't you just accept things as they are?"

And I realize what my answer should have been: "How would you feel if you found out you were denying your son something that could be life-changing?"

19

PAY ATTENTION (2013)

CARTER THARP'S STORY AS TOLD TO JAMIE REESE

W hy do you want to write a story about me? Autism is not that big of a deal.

I feel like I am inside a little white box writing all my thoughts and feelings with dry erase marker, but no one can find me to understand what I am going through. I erase those thoughts and feelings myself, but some things I write in permanent marker, and they will never be forgotten.

If you could come inside, you would see the conversations I've had with you, the experiences I've shared, and the journey of my life; you would understand me.

But I cover what I do not want you to see.

I put away what I do not want lost. *I'll tell you if you let me, though.*

They may not matter to you. *But they matter to me.*

The secrets of my mind are my secrets and not for you to know.

I don't tell you because I don't see you understanding anyway.

You think you do, but you really don't.

It is hard for me to look you in the eye, even harder to be around you. Try learning when people talk so fast and think even quicker. You don't have the patience to wait for my response. Instead, you avoid my words as if I should know to say what you want me to say. This overwhelms me.

I'm going to open this white box for a moment.

The first thing people notice about me is that I'm quiet.

I'm quiet because I don't know what to say.

I see people in a group and I watch them talk to each other.

Their lips move, laughter erupts, and their eyes brighten at the thought of the next word they are going to say.

Instead of words coming to my mind to join their conversations, I watch them and think about their words.

When they turn to me to join, my mind becomes blank.

Everyone I know is an extrovert.

They know what to say.

I don't know how I'm like other kids with autism. I wish I knew more about autism.

I know that I am not like normal kids because I'm quiet.

They can pedal a bike! They can lie. If you want me to lie, forget it.

The main difference between me and normal kids is that they are outgoing—some are loud, but I ignore those kinds of kids. I love my mom, dad grandma, and grandpa, and my uncles. They are my favorite people.

Being overwhelmed is the worst feeling ever. It makes

my brain get dizzy and causes the noises to get louder. It gets on my nerves. Teachers could help by not over-whelming me.

The perfect school would have three floors and a big pool. Teachers wouldn't give a lot of homework; more importantly, they would get to the point. The only classes that would be at that school are Cooking and Science.

Science is the best class. Well, the experiments with chemicals and animals are.

The stupid work is my weakness.

There was this boy who puked on the playground. Five of us were surrounding him and he puked. We picked on him. Well, I don't know if we picked on him or bullied him. I hope he is okay. I feel bad, but I kind of don't because he picked on me too. *I bullied to survive.*

I have a village I created on Mine Craft. The hideout is Hatzan camp. The bandits lurk around in the corners. I've created secret rooms and passageways deep underground so they can't find my treasures and livestock. The fort is called Alatak. It has an escape path. I'm building a new fort. I think I have a good shot at being a game designer when I grow up.

Sure, I have to try harder to learn. Multiple choice tests are not clear. If my grades were based on homework, I'd probably get all A's. My mom helps me through it, but she pushes me and makes me work hard. *She always judges my writing.* When I do my homework wrong, she is there to help me get it right.

At least I am not confused about what she wants. Teachers, on the other hand, are not clear. I ask a question about the assignment and they answer me quickly and get back to being busy.

Something a little weird about me is that I don't go out a lot. It feels normal to be home.

I don't think anyone knows I have autism when they first meet me. If you try to have a conversation with me, you will realize I am quiet and think about things differently than you do. At night I curl up with my weighted blanket and bury my head to get comfy.

What do you need to know about autism?

If kids with autism are like me, then here is what you should know:

People shouldn't talk like stories. Be more plain. Come out with it. Stop being confusing.

Stimming helps me when I am overwhelmed. I tap the plastic hanger against my legs, arms, and sometimes my chin. I also hit it against the back of furniture, which has caused some damage to our couch. If I can't use my hanger, then I walk and pace. You might find me gently tapping myself as if I had the hanger. I chew gum. When I get home though, I get my hanger. I do it when I want, but only at home.

I love to be close to you. It makes me feel safe and to understand you better. I also like to be touched. I used to get my skin brushed, though not so much anymore. I still like it though.

Don't think I have forgotten something just because I don't talk about it; I remember.

I know what right and wrong is. I am like everyone else in that area. *In reality, I'm better at it.*

If you're autistic, you should get a stick or a hanger and try stimming. It will help you.

All right, I think we're done. I like being heard, but I feel overwhelmed.

20

MINE (2013)

CHRISTINE WEIDA'S STORY AS TOLD TO CHRIS BAVENDER

People often ask me if—knowing what I know now—would I have chosen to have children.

My answer never changes.

Yes.

Even though all three of my children have autism.

Yes.

Even though there are no breaks, you just have to keep going. You learn to live without sleep. My husband's job takes a lot of time—sometimes 65 hours a week—so, it's Mom all of the time.

Yes.

Even with all of the challenges. And there are plenty.

My oldest, Jacob, was born on Halloween in 1996. The chord was wrapped around his neck and he was slightly jaundiced, but his APGAR scores were good. He developed fairly normally—sat up, rolled over, and was walking by age one. He was speaking a little, but had difficulties with sleep patterns.

It was in March of 1999—shortly before Jacob's third birthday—that I received the news Jacob had autism. I remember sitting there in disbelief. This is my child—I had all these plans for him and I had to just chuck it all away and start over and not have any expectations.

It's heartbreaking. It really is. Especially when you are told there is nothing you can do. I was told I needed to enroll him in a developmental preschool and that physical and speech therapy was recommended. I was told to fence the yard so he couldn't run away—like they were talking about a dog, not my son.

When I was pregnant with my second child, Violet, my husband, Mike, and I asked the doctor if she was going to have autism as well. We were told there was a good chance she wouldn't since she had a different biological father (I divorced Jacob's dad in 1998).

It didn't matter to me anyway because I knew I would not—could not—abort my baby.

At first, I didn't think she was autistic; she was progressing normally except for her speech. I mentioned something to her doctor who said I was imagining it and Violet was probably just mimicking her brother.

Fourteen months later, Eleana was born. Like the other two, she progressed normally physically. I never really suspected autism with her except for her extreme defiance, lack of speech, and that none of the children seemed interested in playing with each other.

Violet and Eleana both were diagnosed at the same time in May 2006. This time, however, I was a little more prepared for the diagnosis.

But it doesn't mean it's not a daily struggle.

All three children are in public school in Muncie. Eleana is in a mild class, Violet is completely mainstreamed, and Jacob is in a severely disabled class.

Jacob is pretty non-verbal all the time. He gets into a rage at the drop of a hat for no reason; lots of times without warning. He bit me once, just barely breaking the skin, but bruising my arm. I ended up in the hospital with streptococcus toxic shock syndrome. They had to cut out several parts of my arm and all my organs were shutting down—I almost died from my wound.

I don't know what to do with him sometimes. We know he will have to eventually go to a group home for the rest of his life—especially if something were to happen to us. But, as long as we can handle him, we are going to keep him at home. I am *not* going to throw him away or lock him up.

There are days I mourn the child who could have been. But we have to get over it because he is here and this is taking place—this is our life.

Occasionally, I go into the bathroom and lock the door and cry—some days more than others. But I have to be strong for everyone else.

Violet also has an anxiety disorder and is very sensitive. When her brother gets upset, she does, too. She can be really cute—like the time I asked why she waited so long to talk. She told me it was because she had too many questions to ask and didn't know which to ask first.

Eleana is extremely stubborn—especially when she wants something and isn't given it. She literally stands in front of you screaming and doesn't move until she gets what she wants. She will destroy anything at will, especially a freshly cleaned space.

You have to keep Eleana next to you, or at least know where she is and what she is doing, at all times or she will take off—or things will be moved, colored on, cut, ripped. She demands all attention.

It's hard. Very hard.

Schedules are always a challenge; each child has their own time frame and ways of completing tasks. Jacob, you have to physically prompt or take his hand to make him complete a task. Violet and Eleana are a little easier to motivate with a reward.

Discipline is no easy task either; sending them to their room to calm down, or siting them on a chair doesn't always work. We have to be a bit more creative. Taking their favorite thing away for a while and having to listen to all the complaining and whining is trying.

Having "normal" friends hasn't been very easy. Violet is always trying to make friends, but their parents don't want them to spend time with her outside of school. That makes me sad because she thinks no one loves her.

But I do. I love all my children.

People often ask me what I think led to my children being autistic. Was it the vaccinations? The environment?

I think that all plays into it, but no one can prove anything.

You just have to deal with what you see.

And what I see are my children.

21

ASK (2013)

DANA WILLIAMS'S STORY AS TOLD TO CLARISSA CHESLYN

A sk. Ask why she doesn't always make eye contact. Ask why she doesn't scream when a spider scampers across her dinner plate, like most any person would. Ask why she sometimes repeats every word you say. It's echolalia, in case you were curious.

Please don't just look at me and think: *What's wrong with that child?*

I assure you there is nothing wrong with her. Stella is the funniest, most interesting person I have ever met, and she's only three years old.

Every single day with Stella is a joy, an adventure, and a challenge that I am eager to meet—but not a challenge in the way you might think. Each day I am faced with the task of expanding my own mind so that I can see the world around me in the way that she does.

As just one example of the amazing ways my world view has changed: Stella sees words as sounds, not individual letters with individual sounds like T-R-E-E. When she sees the word tree, it's almost like she sees it as a picture of a sound rather than four different sounds put together which is "different," not "wrong." Imagine a world where you are consistently being challenged to see the world through a child's eyes.

I'll let you in on a secret: it's amazing!

It's just one of the amazing things you see when you choose to look at autism as a difference rather than a disability.

In recent years, people have really been emphasizing the idea of tolerance and acceptance when it comes to race, sexuality, and religion. The increase in bullying among school age kids has prompted parents to rally around their kids and raise them to be proud of their individuality—but for some reason developmental disorders have remained attached to their negative stigmas.

Whose disorder is Stella's autism? Hers? Or ours?

Isn't it our responsibility as parents to get to know our own child and figure out what works best for her in terms of how she learns? Author Paul Collins said, "Autists are the ultimate square pegs, and the problem with pounding a square peg into a round hole is not that the hammering is hard work; it's that you're destroying the peg."

When I tell people Stella has autism, their response is often, "I'm sorry." A hush tends to fall over the conversation, and suddenly every bit of eye contact is tainted with a hint of sadness.

I'm not sorry, and I'm not sad.

Nothing bad happened to Stella the day she was diagnosed. She remained the same as she had always been. I felt sad when I heard that my child may struggle, but my worry never came from a place of regret or bitterness toward autism; it was simply that I feared we wouldn't be able to understand each other.

In the seven months since her diagnosis, it has become apparent that while there are many things in the world neither of us will ever understand—we understand each other.

What parent doesn't fear the struggles their child will face? I consider myself lucky to have a child with struggles that can be identified. I am grateful that we have proven ways to help her.

What many people see on the outside as a struggle, I see as a blessing—my beautiful girl whose everyday successes never go unnoticed.

I've been given the opportunity to work with amazing professionals that spend their entire day helping Stella communicate effectively, and helping me understand her. Isn't that kind of a gift?

Yes, there are trials that come with having a child with autism, but there are also amazing triumphs to celebrate. And we spend a lot of time celebrating Stella! Some days will be good and some days will be bad; it's a fact of life not exclusive to autism.

If I could make three wishes for Stella's future, it wouldn't be for a cure or a magic drug to take away her unique traits that came with her autism. My first wish would be for Stella to find her perfect stride, marching to her own drummer. My second wish would be for people to express their curiosity with their words rather than their sideways glances. And my third wish would, of course, be for more wishes.

Stella is my child, and she should be known as a whole, unique, funny, fearless, beautiful child and not a disability or a disorder.

22

OUR UPHILL BATTLE WITH AUTISM (2021)

THE PETERSON'S STORY AS TOLD BY AMBER PETERSON

Our family is complex and may seem unconventional.

But we are trying to overcome many of the same experiences as other families, except we hit an overwhelming lottery of emotions that comes along with raising children with special needs.

We work hard to ensure our family is safe, loved, and appreciated for who they are and the accomplishments they achieve. My husband Kevin and I have been married for sixteen years. We were not prepared for anything needed to raise a child with autism, let alone two. Since we were learning as we were living it, there were extremely trying times causing us to question if we were doing anything right. When the kids were little, I would stop in my tracks and cry at random times.

One of the toughest obstacles to overcome is disagreement over how to raise the kids. It can be stressful and overwhelming, but we push through and do the best we can to prepare the kids for life without us. We are very blessed to have an extended family that is supportive and accepting of the challenges we face. Mom lives with us and has been such a tremendous help over the years giving me the opportunity to take a breather and recharge.

Evan, our youngest, is thirteen and was diagnosed with autism at age two, and then about three years later he was diagnosed with ADHD. He sometimes becomes aggressive and will kick or break objects when he feels intense emotions. His aggressive behavior intensifies when he is very tired and stressed, or when he has anxiety or becomes overwhelmed with emotion. The majority of his behaviors stem from sensory issues, especially with sound. The dog's barking is a major trigger. He wears sound muffling headphones most of the time and even wears them at night while sleeping.

He is very verbal and will let you know what is in his mind and has wonderful conversations with you. He loves YouTube and has his own page where he uploads videos and chats with friends who have the same interest. He is so excited when he gets a new subscriber. He now has 500. He is highly creative and very bright academically and loves to learn new facts about everything. He goes through phases where he becomes fixated on certain topics or objects. Past interests are tornado sirens, car logos, ceiling fans, and regular fans. Did you know there is a ceiling fan museum in Indiana? We went and that was an interesting trip. He loved it.

Patrick, our oldest, is fifteen. He was a preemie weighing only 2lbs, 10oz. That was a very eventful pregnancy. He was diagnosed with autism at age two. Most of his meltdowns were when he was eleven and younger. Those years were incredibly tough. One difficult day he kicked my windshield and cracked it. That was stressful to say the least. The younger years consisted of non-stop screaming, crying, and tearing things up along with the interventions and biomedical treatment we implemented; including a gluten-free, casein-free (GFCF) diet, B-12 shots, supplements, First Steps, ABA, and more.

I researched and learned as much as I could about autism and what the next step in our journey would be. Given all of this, when they meet milestones and goals or do something great it's a party of excitement and celebration.

Patrick is verbal but does not talk a lot. We engage and prompt him first since sometimes it takes longer for him to process what he wants to say. However, despite this, he is very verbal when he chooses to be and asks tons of questions. He likes to joke and prank others. He also enjoys YouTube, reciting and acting out the videos he watches. He is our explorer going outside, looking at trees, digging in the dirt, and taking walks. However, if there is something he is not supposed to do he will do it. He fixates on fans and motors. He lays in front of the fridge and listens. Like his brother he needs sensory input; therefore, he likes to start the washer and watch it spin. In the past he would turn the thermostat off and on to hear it click, then putting his ear on the vent to hear it kick on.

Patrick went through a phase of playing with lighters, so we had to watch him very closely because he is sneaky. Then he decided to cut open all the full pop cans. That was a sticky mess.

He likes to learn, so he will ask questions about everything. He asks tons of "why" questions and repeats them frequently.

I wonder what he will be into next because I may need to prepare.

He is also so funny. He likes jokes and doing things that make other people laugh. One time he came out of the bathroom and shook his butt at us laughing hysterically.

We have had serious issues with meltdowns over the years resulting in aggression and destruction of property. Great news though, since they have gotten older and started medication and therapies, we rarely encounter a meltdown anymore. So, rock on! I have lost track of how many iPads, TVs, and iPhones we have gone through.

We are finally at the point in our lives where Patrick and Evan have matured so much; they are starting to catch up to their typical peers developmentally. Yet they've kept their unique quirks and beautiful personalities.

Since they are teenagers, I am starting the transition process. I'm nervous about it because I want to get it right; making sure they can function in society and live happy, productive lives. Occasionally I worry. I wonder what they would do if I weren't here, so I try to work harder to prepare them for the future.

But teenagers do not make things easy.

We now have time to focus on other things. Therefore, when I can, I share my knowledge, training, personal experience, and resources with families. Having a child with special needs is difficult and with autism there is so much to learn as you go. Over the years I have done extensive autism research, attended conferences and seminars, volunteered, presented at conferences and on panels, and completed many trainings. I hope to ease the stress of families with the knowledge and experience I have acquired. Because of this passion, I have created Instagram and Facebook pages to share resources that families can benefit from.

We are not alone on this journey. Remember to utilize others who have experiences to help you on your journey.

This is just a short snippet into our lives, and we have so many stories and experiences to share. Autism has brought us joy and pain; despite this, we would not have it any other way. However, I could use more sleep! Our children are so unique in their own way, and they are my greatest gifts. They make me laugh, they make me cry, and they make me extremely proud. They are so strong and brave while overcoming and moving forward with all the obstacles set before them.

Temple Grandin once said, "If you've met one person with autism, you've met one person with autism." This quote rings true to individuals with autism and their parents. So, remember to never compare your children's accomplishments or developmental milestones to their peers'. They are on their own journey and have their own hurdles to leap, and their own accomplishments to reach.

The greatest gift you can give them is to be their support system, their rock, and their number one fan because they need you more than they can express. They may not be able to say it or show you, but they love you, need you, and appreciate you. You are their advocate and their voice, so stay strong, take care of yourselves, and enjoy the positive, happy moments and milestones of life.

23

FINDING MY TRUE CALLING (2013)

DIANE'S STORY AS TOLD TO CATHY SHOUSE

Most of my life I knew I wanted to teach special education to children with special needs. Over a 20-year career, I loved each year taught. I enjoyed each child I had in my classroom, even amongst the challenges, my students, staff and parents were the best!

To coin a probably overused cliché: I thrived on "making a difference."

But something was missing. I received children into my classroom that often had previous teachers, techniques, and related services before they reached me. Although my teaching assistants and I scaffolded on the goals and behavior plans that other outstanding disciplines had set the previous school year, I started to feel I was missing a piece of the puzzle. I finally realized it was the history with these children. I wanted to be a part of the journey at the beginning, not somewhere in the middle.

This missing puzzle piece nagged me so much that in 2008, I returned to Ball State University and earned a

Master's degree in Special Education with certification in autism. Autism Spectrum Disorder can be life altering to families, but encouraging in another way as research is revealing more about the cause of autism and treatments available.

With my graduate degree in hand, I left teaching in the public schools and began to work as an early interventionist —also known as a Developmental Therapist or DT—for children with special needs from birth to the age of three through a federally funded program. I thought: *This was it! This is what I should have been doing for the past twenty years!*

As a DT, each day is different, depending on the needs of the children. I usually visit seven or eight of my kiddos per day. I drive to their house, knock on the family's door, and am ushered into the child's environment. For young children with autism, delivering services within their natural environment—wherever they spend the majority of their day—sets the bar for success. For most families, this is the home environment. For some, this could be with a caregiver at a day care or preschool facility.

I bring a large colorful bag with me into each family's home. It is full of toys and materials designed to help facilitate the goals set for each child. Toys can be used to teach play skills and promote social engagement. Special books and puzzles are intended to encourage language skills. Sensory boxes are to help increase tolerance for a variety of texture mediums.

I enjoy working with parents and caregivers; they know their child the best. From their input, I can create materials and strategies that we can work on during a visit, and families are able to continue to work on those for the rest of the week in a variety of different settings. For the child that is recognizing objects in pictures, we can work as a team to create a set of photos that a young one can choose in order to communicate a request for a cookie or a drink. This gives an alternative for a child to make choices while we continue to work on expressive vocabulary.

Studies have revealed that early intervention services can make a positive impact in the areas of communication and social skills with a young child demonstrating characteristics of autism. The Modified Checklist for Autism in Toddlers (M-CHAT) is a screening tool that can be easily used for assessing young children under the age of 30 months to determine a risk for autism. Some health professionals will administer this assessment during pediatric visits with families when autism may be suspected. It would be ideal if all health care providers would include this as part of routine visits.

I do not have all the answers when it comes to working with toddlers with autism. I am so fortunate that I work with such a great team which always includes the families, parents and/or caregiver, but often will include speech, occupational and physical therapists. We can troubleshoot and strategize together to work towards the success of a child's goals. The bonus of it all is when a small child with autism begins to connect with a family member over a shared activity, a social routine, a smile or hug.

Other bonuses are when the child comes to sit in a lap and begins to communicate or when I get to laugh, listen, and yes, shed a tear, with parents about the joys and concerns they have for their little ones.

Autism can often shake the core of a family when the

diagnosis touches their child. It can be a difficult road and different for every family. Something we work on together is understanding that a parent's precious little girl or boy is still that very same child as they were before the diagnosis was delivered.

It is a privilege to work with all kiddos and their families. It is much more than a job; it is my passion.

24

ALL I CAN GIVE (2013)

HALEY CARTER'S STORY AS TOLD TO TIFFANY ERK

You know, some people think that you are valuable based on your ability to work, or what you can contribute or if you can earn an income, but we believe that—because you are alive—you have value. So, it doesn't matter if all six of my children will grow up and leave the home at age eighteen, go on to college, and build a career. They are here for a reason, and I am blessed to be a part of their time here. This life is but a moment, a flash, on the spectrum of eternity.

I have six children, two girls and four boys. Three of my boys are on the spectrum and the youngest is just a baby so we just don't know yet. Two have been diagnosed with autism and a third who is on the spectrum but not yet fully diagnosed, and I think people expect me to mourn that as though it's a great tragedy. What they don't understand is that my children are gifts from God—they are special and unique and I learn from them every day.

It's not easy, though. I never said it was easy. I am diapering, cooking, cleaning, shopping, and home schooling my oldest children from the moment I wake until the moment my head hits the pillow. Our house is loud and unpredictable and chaotic. My husband and I joke that the kids are like popcorn at the dinner table. They jump up and down. First here, now there. Meanwhile, my daughters have to sit quietly, and it is a constant process to explain to them that their brothers can't control their behavior in the same way, so the expectations are different.

My sons' keep me busy—like when they continually remove all of the socks from the dresser and line them up on the floor. Outings are a whole other ball of wax! My son Kaleb learned at a very young age, about two or so, where we were going when we were driving in the car. I didn't know where my parents were driving at that age! But Kaleb did. And when he didn't like where we were going, he would let me know. It finally became part of the routine that I would know that when we got to a particular stoplight he would always begin to scream, so we would talk about our route on the way to the stoplight. And that's what you do. You adjust, and you constantly work with them on behavior modification.

The world sees my sons as different and to other people that means they are defective or they need to be fixed, but truly they are beautifully and wonderfully made, and they should be appreciated and celebrated for who they truly are. I think that when people think about autism, they think about the differences like the vocalizations. When we are in public and my sons will suddenly let out a long "eeeee," people will stare. What I don't think they see or understand is the sweet side of autism.

One hot, summer afternoon, my youngest son's soccer team was posing for a picture. Well, posing is a loose term here. The team ranged in age from 3-4 so they were mostly squirming and jumping up and down, looking around, pretty much everything but sitting still and posing. Parents and coaches were helping and attempting to wrangle the children in their appropriate places. After quite some time of this going on, the photographer was beginning to get frustrated. My son, who didn't understand why we were sitting still in one place for so long, suddenly leaped up and gave the photographer a giant hug. Before the photographer had a chance to compose herself or respond, the entire rest of the team followed suit and, in an instant, the photographer was buried in giggling, cuddling children. Her frustration turned to laughter as she told us nothing like that had ever happened to her before.

And, you know, it's these moments that I see as a mother and as a woman of faith that I want the people who stare at us in public to see, so they can understand these children are truly gifts from God, and they are a part of God's plan for my life. And how lucky am I? I am truly blessed to be able to raise these children that look at the world and interpret it in a completely different way than you and me. Do I get tired? Yes. Do I get frustrated? Yes! But my faith moves me forward. I give my family everything I have to give, all day, every day, and I wouldn't change a thing.

25

CHANGING NORMAL (2013)

KIM MCWHIRT'S STORY AS TOLD TO PAT BENNETT

I didn't learn that my daughter, who is now twelve, had autism until she was about four years old. My pregnancy with her was very difficult and I had to have a C-section. Her brother is three years older that she is, and I was determined not to compare my children to each other. During her early years I was also in the midst of divorcing her father, so I think I was in a kind of fog trying to cope.

When I look back on those early years, I realize that she was doing lots of things that didn't seem normal. She wouldn't look me in the eye, didn't talk much at all, and wasn't potty trained by the time she was four. The thing I really noticed was that she would put her Barbie dolls in a straight line and didn't play with them. She just liked lining them up.

My ex-mother-in-law and sister-in-law were the ones who got my attention and said they suspected she might have autism. I called the Delaware County Special Ed Co-Op and they assessed her. They had a meeting with me, gave me her evaluation, and said they believed she fell on the autism spectrum but was high functioning.

My heart was heavy when I heard that diagnosis knowing that our life would be different from then on. Our normal was changing. My ex just wasn't on the same page as I was and had trouble dealing with it. He seemed to fall off the radar.

I enrolled her in Huffer day care. I was thrilled. I knew she would get the help she needed. Things started improving very quickly after she started. I still have a portfolio from that time showing all the improvements. They sent a note home one day and said I didn't have to send pull-ups anymore; she was potty trained. And where she once just drew lines, she was writing letters. It was like she had been locked in a body that wouldn't co-operate, and their guidance and teaching unlocked her.

I became very proactive during that time. I did a lot of research online on autism and tried to keep up with all the latest information. I also was involved with Interlock, a support group for parents. That was very helpful.

She was still doing unusual things like arm flapping, which she finally stopped, only to switch to picking at her front legs when she was stressed. She still does that. When she was small, she would just eat one color of food, and now she will just eat strange combinations. I think it has something to do with colors and textures, but I don't know. We don't do any special diet therapy. I tried some, and they didn't seem to do anything.

They developed an Individual Educational Plan when she first started school and mainstreamed her. Speech was her main issue, so she worked with a speech therapist and an occupational therapist on physical skills. The schools have been wonderful. I was always busy trying to keep her mind engaged. I just believe it is important to keep kids with autism stimulated. I would read stories to her and talk to her a lot.

Now she is twelve, and she is a really good student and gets all A's. She is very good in Math, and it boggles my mind because I am not very good at it. I am very proud of her. The hard thing for me now is to see her alone and not doing things with a lot of friends, but then she is very comfortable alone. I am more of a social butterfly, and so I struggle more with her aloneness than she does.

She and her brother get along well, but sometimes she says things that aren't appropriate and it is frustrating for him. I hope he feels that I have given him lots of attention even though she has special needs. I would be heartbroken if I thought he didn't feel that way. I am not totally comfortable either when we are in social situations because I can't anticipate what she might do or say in each different situation. I just want her to be accepted. I have never used her autism as an excuse and have always told that to her teachers and our family.

She was involved in the BSU Prism project for special needs kids and she has a beautiful voice. She sang a solo. She is such a good student but has difficulty with reading comprehension, and I worry about that as she gets older. I am also a little worried because lately she zoned out on a weekend when she was very stressed. I don't know what that means at this point. I want to read more on the brain so I can understand what is going on. As she is getting older, I am trying to find a balance between letting her be herself and yet helping her do things that will keep her engaged and accepted.

I am afraid her brain will revert back if I don't keep her involved.

I volunteered to tell our story because I knew I wanted to help others as soon as I found out she had a type of autism. I have kept all my materials and am always willing to share. I would tell other parents to get involved with a support group of other parents because that helped when she was younger. I think it is very important to stay involved and to learn as much as you can. You also have to be proactive with doctors so that they really understand what is going on.

I am lucky because my present husband treats her as his own and is understanding, and my mom is the one I call when I get frustrated. She has always been there for me. At the present, I wish there was a group for parents of teens because it is harder to help them and yet give them space to be themselves.

As she gets older, I want to continue learning about the brain and find some kind of work related to that.

26

ON HER OWN (2021)

KIM MCWHIRT'S STORY AS TOLD TO DANIELLE
WASSON

S o much life has been lived in the years since I first
shared about Madison and her story in *Facing
Autism.*

Nine years ago, I shared her story because other parents
and their stories were a huge source of strength on my journey. I wanted to be that for other parents that found themselves figuring out how to best care for their autistic child.

Early in Madison's life she received excellent aid in the
schools she attended. Nine years ago, she was twelve and
receiving straight A's in school. She continued on and was
mainstreamed with her peers.

As Madison excelled with her grades, she did find other
aspects of school challenging. She struggled making a
connection with the other students. Socially connecting
and reading someone's body language continues to be an
aspect of autism that is frustrating. She would find herself
alone in independent activities. When Madison did connect
with peers, she tended to be in very intense relationships;

ultimately resulting in a fall out for misunderstanding in body language and communication. Today, this continues to be her biggest struggle, and so she continues to try and learn to be like others.

Madison learned to advocate for herself early on. She found an opportunity to connect with a teacher once a day to destress. She also knew when it was best for her to transition to a different school. After attending Monroe and Muncie high schools, she told me she had made arrangements to finish out her high school career at the Excel Center. Maybe I babied her too much those first years of high school, but I couldn't help but agree to her wishes.

In 2019, Madison graduated with her Core 40 diploma. I was so proud!

Next, Madison attended Anderson University living on campus. Unfortunately, when COVID hit she had to attend classes online and this became quite a struggle. Madison then transferred to Marian University and has now landed at Ball State. She will start online classes the second semester.

Madison has had a few different jobs, and each shares a theme of wanting to care for others. At Ball State she plans to study in the ABA Therapy program. I strongly encourage her to stay on this path. I firmly believe she can help those students and their families since she was once in their shoes.

As she has before, Madison continues to advocate for herself. She found her own apartment over a year ago and decided to call Kokomo, Indiana home. I enjoy having Madison drive me around Kokomo and watching her navigate. I'm proud of the way she has truly made the city her home; knowing all the backroads and having that level of self-assurance.

In her free time, Madison enjoys computer games and picking different television series to follow on Netflix. She takes such pride in following the storyline. The *Law and Order* series has been one of her favorites.

In my original story I shared that Madison's father struggled to connect with her, and that is still true today. I've remarried, and Madison has only allowed the bond to go so far. I'm thankful that Madison and her brother do have a good relationship. I think having Madison as a sister has made my son a very accepting human being. He has always had a big heart, and growing up with Madison has taught him tolerance and patience.

I'm proud of Madison and all of her independence. Graduating high school, living on her own, and now attending college were all things I wasn't sure would be a reality for Madison. She has overcome so many obstacles.

If I could go back to the moment when Madison was diagnosed and give my younger self advice, I'd say: "Life goes on. She will succeed. There will be setbacks. Relax and enjoy the moment because the future comes anyway."

27

BEING THE KEY (2013)

LISA COMBS'S STORY AS TOLD TO ABBY WALTON

I first heard the word autism in the early 1980s while sitting in a classroom at Ball State University. I went to Ball State to study marketing, but it wasn't really me so I went through a series of majors including deaf education. It was during one of my special education classes where I first learned about autism. My professor showed a movie titled *Sonrise*, which followed the life of a young autistic boy. I'll never forget watching the screen and being drawn to the look in that child's eyes. What I saw was a child who had thoughts and feelings, but couldn't get them out. It was as if he was locked inside of himself. It was during that class I decided to help families unlock the mysteries of autism.

After class, I went up to my professor and told him I wanted to specialize in autism. I'll never forget his response. He told me that I wouldn't want to specialize in *that* because I would never see a child with autism in my classroom. At the time, the prevalence of children with autism was about one in ten-thousand. And when a child was diagnosed, he or she would be put into a special school and never really given an education. Although I wasn't receiving any encouragement, I knew I was supposed to learn more about autism. Bit by bit, I was starting to become that key that could help families turn that autism lock.

After Ball State, I went on to teach mild-mentally handi-capped kids in Indianapolis. I'll always remember this one kid named Tyler. He was a third grader and no one really knew how to categorize him. He could read at grade level, but had some very strange social skills. One day he came in from recess and said, "Man, I'm sweating like a corn cob."

Tyler also had this fascination with maps. He could look at a map and tell me how many different route combina-tions there were from my house to the school. I had a feeling this little guy was on the spectrum, but in the late 80s no one was giving kids that label. All they knew was that he was different, and although he probably could have been in a regular class, his abnormalities meant going to school in a self-contained classroom.

After teaching in Indy, I moved to Ohio in the 90s to supervise county and regional special education programs. However, my main focus continued to be learning more about autism. In 2009, I started working for Ohio's Center for Autism and Low Incidence as a regional autism coach. It was during this time that I spoke at several conferences about autism, including strategies to help educators and parents. I found that although educational, a conference really wasn't what these people needed. A teacher would go to the conference, but when he or she got back to the classroom, they wouldn't know how to implement the strategies so nothing would change.

I knew that I needed to help teach others to become keys in their own lives. So, for the past four years, I've been supervising a team that works with educators in Ohio to implement evidence-based practices for students with autism.

I get so passionate when I talk about this because we spend an entire year with teachers helping them learn ways to communicate, and, ultimately, educate these children. People often equate communication with intelligence, but that's not always true.

Remember Tyler? Last Christmas, his mother found my address and sent me a card to tell me that her son had graduated from high school and found a job he enjoyed. It really struck a chord with me because we often look at the challenges facing autistic kids, but often forget about their strengths. It's up to us as teachers and parents to find those strengths within our kids and help drawl them out. That's why I'm so excited about our virtual coaching.

By turning on a computer, iPad or phone, educators and parents, no matter where they live, are able to show me and other coaches what's happening with their kids in real time. For example, a mother recently texted me a video of her young son. The doctors think he may have autism, but since he's so young, they won't fully diagnose him yet. Her message to me was, "What do you think? Is this a sign of autism?"

I looked at the video, and it makes me cry just thinking about it, because what I saw was a child playing with his toys. But, in this mother's mind, every move her child made was another potential sign of autism. However, because I was able to take a look at the video right then, I was able to give her some piece of mind for at least another day. I was able to tell her while he may someday receive an autism diagnosis, today he was just being a normal toddler.

When I first heard about autism, I never could have imagined how much it would change my life and the lives of so many others across the world. From one in ten-thousand to now as high as one in fifty, according to a recent study, it's amazing how far we've come and, yet, how far we still have to go in understanding and treating this disorder.

My life's mission, to unlock the mysteries of autism, began that day at Ball State. By providing services that give live feedback about a child's behaviors, I believe I'm helping create more keys.

And the more keys this world has, the closer we can unlock the thinking, feeling people that live inside our autistic children.

28

DRIVE (2013)

MARIE'S STORY AS TOLD TO J.R. JAMISON

I t started with the virus, when Leslie was three. It had a way of triggering it. She and her dad both got the flu. Viruses have a way of unlocking dormant genes. But I'm not a doctor, so I don't know.

But that's when it all changed.

She started to regress. She stopped her potty training. She started acting out. She started kicking and biting. The kid who was seemingly well-adjusted was gone overnight. She had become a different child in just a couple of months. It was fast.

That was the start of the meltdowns.

Then my marriage fell apart. Her dad was becoming a person he wasn't when we met; he was dealing with his own health issues, and all of these events toppled upon one another—it was the beginning of the end.

We divorced.

Daycares wouldn't take her. I couldn't leave her with any family or friends for an extended period of time. It made it hard to hold down a job. I felt helpless. I just didn't know how to help my kid. I really didn't know what to do, and I had very few resources after the divorce to figure it all out. I had to move into my parents' house for a year. But they became exhausted.

I was able to get a job at a local daycare center. They were great, and I could take Leslie to work with me. There were other kids there for her to play with, and she still had some meltdowns; but there were other staff members who could help me. I wasn't alone.

And then she started school.

The first few years were tough. She'd run out, she'd kick and scream at her teachers, and I was getting calls every other day. I'd cringe when I'd hear the phone ring. I knew it was them calling about Leslie. But despite her behavior, she is brilliant and was placed in the gifted and talented program.

When she was in that program, that's when she got bullied. All of those kids are so smart; they know how to get away with it. But I caught one of the kids bullying her one day with my own two eyes. I couldn't believe it. But then there were the parents of those kids. I never thought I'd get upset saying this . . . it just seemed like all of the kids were picking on her . . . and the adults would just roll their eyes. There was no control. The other kids and their parents stayed away from us. They'd whisper and look in horror. We were rejected by all of the others; that's, that's how it felt. You know that song from Dumbo, "Baby Mine"? I used to sing it to Leslie to ease the pain . . . to ease my pain. I don't think she ever knew the real meaning behind the song, but for me, I could relate.

They eventually kicked her out of the program. The teacher said Leslie was too stressful for her, and she didn't belong. Leslie's behavior was awful, I get it, but that teacher just wasn't willing to adjust or willing to reach her. Isn't that a teacher's job?

She kept a journal on Leslie. Everything she did—her meltdowns. How did the teacher even have time? She didn't do it to be helpful; she did it to prove a point to me that my child was out of control. That wasn't helpful.

We were referred to Ball State counseling. We were assigned a doctoral student. He was nice, but clearly still learning. I shared the teacher's journal with him, but after hours and days of observing Leslie, he determined there was nothing wrong.

Then her pediatrician referred us to Riley. She felt that Leslie had been sexually abused. She wanted an exam. I took her to Riley and had to put my seven-year-old daughter through all of that—when I knew she hadn't been abused—for them to tell me she hadn't. That's when the doctors determined that we might be dealing with autism.

A few months later, as Leslie entered the second grade, she was finally diagnosed with Asperger's.

———

There's a relief in knowing; all of those years of not knowing, we finally had an answer. The doctors wanted to start medication immediately. I refused. To this day Leslie doesn't take medication for her Asperger's.

She's adjusted well over time. We've still not told the school system and don't plan to do so. Labels can create a divide. Not just with other students, but it puts a stigma on her that teachers can't fail to recognize.

Now as a teenager, she has some kids who pick on her, but she doesn't get it. It bounces off of her; she's in her own universe. That's good, I guess. Very few things affect her, good or bad, but I want her to build deep relationships with people.

Most of her relationships are with inanimate objects. It's taken me awhile to adjust to that. But that's her world. She's obsessed with anime, Japan, all of it. She doesn't get social cues; and she'll talk about a topic more than people would like to hear. But that's part of it. Her Pokémons are an extension of her. She takes them to school, but the rule is that they have to stay in her locker.

She has friends. They're all either Asperger's or ADHD. They naturally gravitate toward each other. It's just natural because they have so much in common. Like Leslie, most of the high functioning kids aren't labeled through the school system.

———

I do worry about her independence. She wants to go to college. She's brilliant and would excel; I have no doubt she'd make a great scientist or artist. But she would go days without showering if I didn't prompt her. She hoards. It's part of it. She can't let go of inanimate objects because of the relationships she develops with things. Her room is a mess, beyond just teenager messy. I worry what life will be like for her on her own, away at college.

She's supposed to get her license in a year. That worries

me. Not just as a parent, but it worries me to think about her behind the wheel of a car. But she wants to drive, and it's a rite of passage, so I'm still considering the options.

But college?

I don't know. I think she can make it, but we need to take it one day at a time. She might really surprise us all.

Let's focus on the driving first.

29

FOR THE LOVE OF GWYN (2021)

AMANDA ROBERTS'S STORY AS TOLD TO SONYA PAUL

"God grant me the serenity to accept the things I cannot change."

I pray the Serenity Prayer on hard days as I raise my autistic daughter, Gwyn.

I walk through the worst of it all and prepare myself for what lies ahead in the future. I spend time looking for the positivity, courage, and strength in loving her.

When Gwyn is mad or upset, we all pay for it in some way; most times, me. She pinches, and eventually, she is on to something else and is happy. She trusts me, so I am often the target of her resistance or unhappiness. It does pass.

And despite the physical pain I might suffer on any given day with Gwyn and her moods, God did bless me with Gwyn.

I am a more patient, understanding, and empathetic person. God knew long ago, we belong together; he has designed me through trials and growth to be her mom. There was a plan.

I saw something very different about Gwyn quickly after her birth.

I think in hindsight, I knew from the beginning, but I think being a first-time mom I wasn't sure what I was feeling or seeing. Gwyn is precious and always has been special. But from the beginning it was hard. She never learned to self-soothe, honestly needed to be moving, hardly slept unless being held, only allowed certain people to hold her or love on her (me, her dad, my sister, and my mom). In fact, most everyone else it was a struggle.

She just wasn't comfortable letting people into her circle. She nursed constantly or wanted to. At the time, I just thought she was baby and that sometimes some babies need more than others. But looking back, I see the signs. For example, she always had to have two things in her hands. Constantly. She was doing puzzles for a two-year-old at six months and mastering them quickly. Clearly, Gwyn was not interested in the same things other kids her age were.

And so, it was around fifteen months when I started really thinking things through about my girl. Just something was off. She was not really talking besides a few words, and really had no interest. Her meltdowns were like nothing I had seen before. There was just no consoling her until she was done. During that time though she had ear infections all the time, so I honestly thought some of it was that and it would change eventually.

However, around twenty-one months, she had tubes placed and adenoids removed. Things did not change. That is when I knew for sure. I started reading signs of autism in girls, and I saw Gwyn staring back at me. I just didn't know what to do next. She was in the first steps and I had talked with our family doctor. I finally asked for a specialist referral just after she turned two.

I was able to find a doctor who listened in order to discover the correct diagnosis. And I read everything and researched as much as possible to understand Gwyn. We saw Dr. Escobar just before Gwyn was two-and-a-half, and I felt like I had found a safe place. He asked me if I was familiar with autism and I said, "Yes!" I also told him that if he says it is autism then "great," at least I will be able to start helping her and finding her all she needed.

How to survive daily life in order to reach out to Gwyn is another story. Early on, before any diagnosis, I started realizing Gwyn needed dim lighting, quieter sounds. She didn't like large stores so I didn't force her to do that; she liked to know what to expect so I would tell her multiple times what we were doing, where we were going, the process to get ready and steps to take etc. It was like a broken record, but it worked. I started using sign language with her as well. I never stopped showing her affection and encouraging her to show others and that it was okay. We use sign language daily to communicate. Also, replication is the key. It is an unconditional love. I love Gwyn without any conditions, but, of course, she has her boundaries. We work within her realm.

One realm that Gwyn totally controls is her food intake. Gwyn eats a very little. She used to eat everything, but around age two she started getting more and more restrictive. Now it is very restrictive. She eats the yellow bag of Original Lays Potato Chips, sometimes the red bag of Wavy Chips; Organic White Cheddar Cheese Puffs from Target, in the purple bag; occasionally White Cheddar Popcorn, in the black and yellow bag; Pizza King breadsticks; only Chicken McNuggets from McDonalds, and only when at her dads; occasionally baby Bel Cheeses, the original in the red wrapper; Eggo Toaster Sticks; Goldfish or pretzels (only the little sticks); Doritos; and Triscuits. We cannot use generics; she somehow knows the difference. She must be able to see the bags or boxes. She is unwilling to try anything else. She only drinks water.

It is true, family life changes within a social unit raising an autistic child, and it is also the case with me. Throughout this process of raising Gwyn, I have experienced divorce and dating again, becoming a new blended family—and as a mom, I've changed too.

I have always been someone with high expectations and planning on the future, but having Gwyn and going through this journey with her has forever changed me. I have learned to let go and live in the present. I have gained so much patience, compassion, and understanding. I consistently thank God for blessing me to be Gwyn's mom. I truly believe there was a reason we were paired together. Just as I nourish and help her, she teaches me and helps me evolve into a better human being. I cannot imagine my life without her. Days are unexpected and moments are cherished.

She really loves her stepbrothers too; she is becoming more open to them.

Still, while family get-togethers are a challenge, they are becoming better. For the first four years or so, I could not sit at a dinner table with family. Gwyn just could not handle it. So, I often went off by myself to be with her and ate later. She is getting better with large family gatherings. One thing

I started doing a few years back was to pack a bag of some of her favorite books and dolls etc., and then whenever we get to the gathering, I find her a safe spot where she can go to get away and be alone when she needs. I explain to her it is her safe place. It works really well.

As exhausting and trying as autism can be, I look at all the blessings it brings. Try to find the positives and make it about that and don't stress about the unknown future.

Gwyn is working toward joining an inclusion classroom at West View Elementary. I am looking into getting her into the Autism Kindergarten at East Washington Academy.

In reflecting on how we relax and connect, Gwyn loves playing outside, books, anything regarding water. She loves it.

And she is showing more emotion. Gwyn has become very affectionate. But I truly don't think she would have been if it had not been for me (and her dad) really encouraging her to hug people and sign "love you," etc.—this is really all on her terms. It's Gwyn, it really is, and I am her partner on this path. God grants me the serenity and calm each day to be what she needs in a mother.

30

A BOY'S BEST FRIEND (2021)

ALYSSA BURKHART'S STORY AS TOLD TO BETH MESSNER

Before Ryan came into our lives, our lives were far from normal.

The behaviors triggered by my son Tyler's autism meant we couldn't go anywhere. We constantly walked on eggshells, trying to prevent explosive and dangerous behaviors. I never knew how long I could go to the grocery without Tyler flipping out and we would have to leave. He would get kicked out of school because of behavioral meltdowns. At one point, the doctors told us that because of Tyler's behaviors, he likely would end up in jail or a residential home.

Then Ryan joined our family and we were able to lead a more normal life.

Ryan is my son's service dog—a golden retriever with the biggest stinking smile. Ryan came into our lives when Tyler was seven-and-a-half years old. We had been searching for ways to manage Tyler's behavior since he was two-and-a-half. After brain mapping revealed the severity of his condition and potential for life-long struggle, our doctor said Tyler will need to stay calm at all times to prevent his triggers. Because animals help him stay calm, she suggested we get a service dog. When Ryan's trainer finally delivered him to us, Tyler initially was a little unsure: "Can I pet him? Can I hug him?" But Tyler and Ryan bonded very quickly. The trainer said she had never seen such a quick and solid bond. I think that's partly because Ryan thinks he's human, and Tyler often acts like a dog when they play together!

While Tyler is high-functioning, he has difficulty with emotional socialization and has severe dysregulation of his mood and emotions. Ryan helps Tyler address these issues. When Tyler focuses on Ryan, he's less likely to be triggered by stimuli in the outside world; like noises that bother him because of his hypersensitivity to sound. If Tyler has a behavioral episode in a store, we pull him and Ryan off to the side and let Ryan calm Tyler. If Tyler gets a little squirrely in the classroom, a teacher might say, "Hey, why don't you go take Ryan for a walk?" This helps Tyler regain his focus because he is concentrating on caring for his best friend.

My husband and I also noticed that Ryan helps Tyler feel more confident and responsible. For example, Tyler is better able to verbalize when things bother him—"I don't like the lights; they're too bright" or "I don't like the sound," like the clanking of silverware or the buzzing of fluorescent lights. And Tyler has grown a lot by taking care of Ryan. We told him, "This is your dog. So, you get his vest, you get his leash on, you load him in the car, you feed him." And sometimes, if I'm lucky, he'll pick up dog poop. Caring for Ryan has also helped Tyler learn to take initiative and become more independent. He participates in training Ryan and has full control of him as a handler.

Although there are still experiences that would be too overwhelming for Tyler, like going to the State Fair, Ryan enables us to do some of the things that other families do. For example, now we can occasionally go out to eat, travel, and do "normal kid stuff" rather than isolate inside our home. When we go out to dinner, Tyler will finish his meal and climb under the table to sit with Ryan and play on his iPad. This allows my husband and me to enjoy a meal together. We also enjoy camping with our travel trailer several times a year. After doing things like hiking, Tyler can go into the trailer with Ryan to decompress. I have pictures of Tyler and Ryan on their beds together, smiling. Tyler is even able to attend a summer camp with Ryan.

Ryan's presence in our lives has also provided me with many opportunities to help teach others about autism and service animals. That is the reason I started a Facebook page entitled *Adventures of Tyler and Ryan the Autism Service Dog*. The page is mostly for Tyler's teachers and our family and friends. With Tyler's approval, I share stories and pictures of Tyler and Ryan to help explain what their world is like. This helps educate others about why Tyler might need to have alone time or needs to climb under a table in a restaurant, what stimuli might trigger a behavior, or how we respond to certain behaviors.

This page, and our public outings, also enable me to help others understand the role a service dog plays and how to appropriately behave around them. Ryan is cute and friendly—people just gravitate toward him. Some people are polite and ask questions. But there also are people who take pictures or engage in "drive-by petting." They just reach out and start touching Ryan, even though his vest says: *Do not pet.* I mean, service dogs are very clearly marked. When people do that, he gets all excited and it breaks his concentration. That can be very dangerous, especially if Ryan was addressing one of Tyler's behaviors and trying to calm him.

As a nurse-practitioner, I've also provided training for other medical professionals who work with autistic patients. The medical field provides very little training in this area. So, I've created training modules for staff who work in urgent care and with special needs kids. I teach them how to avoid a meltdown and to adjust to their patients' needs. I've also received a grant to make sensory boxes for those patients.

What started as a nightmare, has turned into a blessing. While our lives are far from normal, we have made the most of it and are able to show people that living with autism is not a curse, it can be rewarding.

STORYTELLERS & WRITERS

Bios

Chris Bavender *is a Muncie native and a Ball State University alumna. She has more than 25 years' experience as a print and broadcast journalist, and is a freelance writer for several regional publications. She currently lives in Noblesville and is the Public Affairs Officer for FBI Indianapolis which covers the state of Indiana.*

Pat Bennett *is a retired nurse who taught at the Anderson University School of Nursing for over 25 years. She volunteers with several agencies that work with poverty and persons with brain disorders.*

Liz Bergren *is the Development Director for CROSSROAD Child & Family Services in Fort Wayne, Indiana, and she is a graduate of Ball State University.*

Michael Brockley *has been writing poems since he was a boy with a burr hair cut in Connersville, Indiana. Several of his poems have appeared in Facing Project publications.*

Alyssa Burkhart, *mother to Tyler, is a family nurse practitioner working to educate health care staff and providers to help accommodate the needs of their autistic patients. She has been married to her husband, father of Tyler, for 15 years.*

Haley Carter *is a stay-at-home parent. If you connected with Haley's story, you can reach her at haleyhearing@yahoo.com.*

Jules Carter is a mom who is just finishing up her home-schooling journey with Logan and appreciates learning from the challenges that each day brings.

Logan Carter is getting ready to start college in the fall, loves playing video games with friends and family all over the world, and enjoys seeing local kids get out into nature in the club he started five years ago, Wildlife Warriors Indiana.

Clarissa Cheslyn is a PhD student in Health Communication at Indiana University. In her free time, she enjoys writing and performing acoustic shows around Indianapolis.

Suzanne Clem has been part of the Muncie community since moving to Ball State in 1997 from Monroeville, Indiana. She's been involved with the Smart Living Project, Muncie Young Professionals, Tour of Muncie, church music groups, and likes to be on her bicycle and in her garden. Suzanne is the Vice President of Community Engagement for Open Door Health Services.

Lisa Combs has 35 years of experience as a special educator. She has a Master's Degree in Special Education from Ball State University. She supervises The Miami Valley Autism Coaching Team and also coaches school personnel, parents, families, and individuals with autism through her own consulting practice, Spectrum Autism Solutions: www.specturmautismsolutions.com.

Debbie DuBois is a mother of two daughters and a son, Joel, and a grandmother to two grandkids, Sammy and Sylvia, with whom Debbie loves to play learn and do crafts. Debbie is Joel's strongest advocate and champion.

Joel DuBois is a 22-year-old Personal Computer (PC) Expert. He graduated from high school and attended the Erskine Green Training Institute in Muncie. Joel connects to the world through his parents, his family, his friends, his work, and through his love of all things PC. Joel always says, "Having autism will not hold me back; it might just take me a little longer!"

Dr. Tiffany Erk *is a Muncie native and Ball State University alumna. She is the mother of two teenagers and has been happily married for over twenty years.*

Cameron Hoesman *is one happy young man! He loves listening and singing to music, plus drawing and being in nature!*

Mother of three, **Belinda Hughes**, *is founder and lead clinical consultant at Behavior Associates of Indiana, a clinic she started with the goal of enhancing lives for individuals living with autism spectrum disorders.*

J.R. Jamison *is a founder and president of The Facing Project and co-host of The Facing Project Radio Show on NPR (produced by Indiana Public Radio). His memoir,* Hillbilly Queer, *was released in 2021.*

Darolyn "Lyn" Jones *is mother to a joy boy with disability, an activist, a professor, and a writer. Her purpose in life is to use her words to help advocate and lift up those voices that society doesn't listen to, ignores, dismisses, disregards, doesn't believe in, and doesn't value. Stories humanize us and create space for everyone at life's beautiful and messy table.*

Kim McWhirt *and her husband, Paul, live in Muncie with their two dogs, Bama and Spencer. Kim actively follows autism support groups on social media and updated autism research online.*

Beth Messner *is an Associate Professor of Communication Studies at Ball State University. She teaches courses related to rhetoric and persuasion and also studies the discourse of those whose voices are traditionally silenced.*

Jason Newman *is the CEO of the Boys & Girls Clubs of Muncie.*

Emma Osborn works at IU Health Ball, Blackford, and Jay Hospitals. If you connected with Emma's story, you can reach her on Facebook at www.facebook.com/EmmaIndeed/.

Having children with autism has driven **Amber Peterson** to advocate and research. She has volunteered with organizations, participated in trainings, and educated herself about autism, and she is willing to share her knowledge and personal experiences with the hope of helping families easier navigate their journey. Amber can be reached at autismspecneedsresourcesin@gmail.com; www.autismspecneedsresourcesin.com/; or on Facebook and Instagram: autismspecneedsresourcesin/.

Sonya Paul is an Indiana University Dual Credit, English, Composition, Communications, and Yearbook instructor at Blue River Valley Jr-Sr High School. She has also raised a son with Asperger's.

Jamie Reece is a mother of three by day, and a relentless idealist by night. She is working on her first novel.

Kyle Reninger is the President of Acquisitions at Sea Salt & Cinnamon, an all-vegan bakery located in the heart of downtown Muncie with services in Fort Wayne and Indianapolis.

Christine Rhine is a freelance writer and editor with a background in newspaper reporting and editing. She relishes the power of stories to bring us all closer together.

Amanda Roberts is a stylist and make-up artist at John Jay & Co.

Allison Shelley teaches nursing full time at Ball State University and works in the ICU at Ball Memorial Hospital. She loves hanging out with friends and family, watching crime shows with Jackson, and watching Parker play baseball.

Chad Shelley is the Vice President of Northwest Bank.

Jackson Shelley is a freshman at Muncie Community High

School where he is enjoying learning Japanese. He loves food, traveling, his friends, and his family. He is hoping to pass Drivers Ed this spring and maybe get a job.

Cathy Shouse is a freelance journalist, whose work has appeared in four Indiana newspapers and several magazines—including the Saturday Evening Post. She is the author of Images of America: Fairmount.

Tom Steiner lives in Muncie with his wife, Kristine. When not working as freelance maker or rehabbing his house in the Historic Emily Kimbrough Neighborhood, Tom is always looking for new and interesting challenges.

Madison Stevenson is an individual with autism who has a strong passion for helping other individuals overcome the toughest obstacles and push forward to success in all aspects of their life! Growing up with autism, and making many mistakes along the way, has allowed her to see the improvements that need to be made within herself and her interactions with others; and she has also developed a strong goal to get her PhD and become a Board-Certified Behavior Analyst Doctor (BCBA-D) to help guide others who have been through similar situations and apply her experiences and knowledge to new situations that she has never dealt with. She is currently going to Ball State University to pursue a Bachelor of Science in Applied Behavior Analysis.

Carter Tharp graduated from Muncie Central High School where he was a member of the National Honor Society and a Varsity swimmer for three years. He earned an Associate's Degree Cum Laude in General Studies from Ivy Tech Community College, where he has continued his education in Physical Therapy and will be applying to that program this spring. In addition to his studies, Carter obtained his lifeguard certification and works as a lifeguard during the summers. He continues to thrive and never gives up on his goals.

Annie Timmerman is married to her high school sweetheart, Kelsey, and is called mom by her daughter, Harper, and son, Griffin. She enjoys working in the landscape design department of Wasson Nursery. Annie loves watching Harper play sports and Griffin play piano.

Kelsey Timmerman is a founder of The Facing Project and a New York Times *bestselling author of three books. More importantly he's a dad to Harper and Griffin and a husband to Annie.*

Dennis Lee Tyler is an autism advocate and lover of Muncie. If you connected with Dennis's story, you can contact him at dltyler1980@gmail.com or on Twitter @dennisltyler.

Rebecca Tyler is a Compliance Manager at Ball State University.

Abby Walton has worked in television for the past sixteen years, currently as a News Anchor and Reporter at WCTV Eyewitness News and FOX 49 news in Tallahassee, Florida. A Ball State University graduate and Hoosier native, Walton has worked on numerous stories to educate people about autism spectrum disorder. One of her reports called, "We Exist: Girls and Women Living with Autism," won the 2009 Gracie which is a national award given out by the Alliance for Women in Media.

Danielle Wasson and her husband, Dan, have three children they are raising in Muncie while running the family landscaping business. Dani's mom was a special needs teacher for 30 years and advocating for those with autism is near and dear to her heart.

Christine Weida is a tax preparer and Office Manager at H&R Block. If you were moved by Christine's story, you can contact her at christine_weida@yahoo.com.

Brian White is a devoted Christian who is autistic and a video-game fanatic, and he's a Ball State University graduate.

Dana Williams is a wife, mom, artist, crafter, and seeker of truth and justice. If you connected with Dana's story, you can contact her at danadee74@gmail.com.

Cheryl Williamson is in her 40th year of teaching high school French and English and still enjoying it! The chance to interview parents of an autistic child and writing about it has helped her gain some insight into some of her own students.

SPONSORS

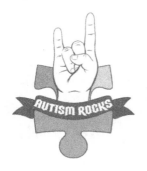

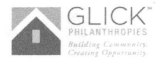

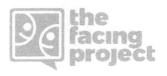

ABOUT THE FACING PROJECT

The Facing Project is a 501(c)(3) nonprofit that creates a more understanding and empathetic world through stories that inspire action. The organization provides tools and a platform for everyday individuals to share their stories, connect across differences, and begin conversations using their own narratives as a guide. The Facing Project has engaged more than 7,500 volunteer storytellers, writers, and actors who have told more than 1,500 stories that have been used in grassroots movements, in schools, and in government to inform and inspire action.

In addition, stories from The Facing Project are published in books through The Facing Project Press and are regularly performed on *The Facing Project Radio Show* on NPR.

Learn more at facingproject.com
Follow us on Twitter and Instagram @FacingProject

CPSIA information can be obtained
at www.ICGtesting.com
Printed in the USA
BVHW031408140422
634340BV00004B/29

9 781734 558180